ATLAS OF
Small animal surgery
THORACIC, ABDOMINAL, AND SOFT TISSUE TECHNIQUES

ATLAS OF
Small animal surgery

THORACIC, ABDOMINAL, AND SOFT TISSUE TECHNIQUES

Richard E. Hoffer, D.V.M., M.S.

Associate Professor of Small Animal Surgery, New York
State Veterinary College, Cornell University; Diplomate,
American College of Veterinary Surgeons

SECOND EDITION

with 319 illustrations in 74 plates and 25 figures
Tone drawings by Ronald Cherkas and George Batik

The C. V. Mosby Company

Saint Louis   1977

SECOND EDITION

Copyright © 1977 by The C. V. Mosby Company

All rights reserved. No part of this book may be reproduced in any manner without written permission of the publisher.

Previous edition copyrighted 1973

Printed in the United States of America

Distributed in Great Britain by Henry Kimpton, London

The C. V. Mosby Company
11830 Westline Industrial Drive, St. Louis, Missouri 63141

Library of Congress Cataloging in Publication Data

Hoffer, Richard E
  Atlas of small animal surgery.

  First published in 1973 under title: Stereoscopic atlas of small animal surgery.
    Bibliography: p.
    Includes index.
    1. Dogs—Surgery. 2. Cats—Surgery. I. Title.
[DNLM: 1. Abdomen—Surgery—Atlases. 2. Animal diseases—Surgery—Atlases. 3. Surgery, Operative—Veterinary—Atlases. 4. Thorax—Surgery—Atlases.
SF911 H698s]
SF991.H58 1977   636.7′08′97   77-3627
ISBN 0-8016-2221-2

TS/U/B 9 8 7 6 5 4 3 2 1

Foreword

It is a pleasure to compose a foreword to Dr. Hoffer's surgical atlas. Dr. Hoffer was associated with Auburn University from 1961 through 1963 in a Master of Science program in surgery. While at Auburn, Dr. Hoffer pioneered in esophageal surgery and modern gaseous anesthetic methods and equipment. His contributions in these areas have been exceptional.

After leaving Auburn University, Dr. Hoffer continued his surgical and educational experiences at the University of Pennsylvania Medical School and the University of Missouri Veterinary College and is currently at New York State Veterinary College at Cornell University in Ithaca, New York. He is a diplomate of the American College of Veterinary Surgeons.

This surgical atlas for small animals has been greatly enhanced by the descriptive accompanying illustrations. Dr. Hoffer's surgically sound methods have been briefly and graphically presented and should be a valuable reference for students and graduate veterinarians. Dr. Hoffer is to be complimented on a most exceptional contribution to veterinary surgical literature.

B. F. Hoerlein

Alumni Professor and Head of the
Department of Small Animal Surgery and Medicine,
Auburn University, Auburn, Alabama

v

Preface TO SECOND EDITION

The *Atlas of Small Animal Surgery* has been republished without the stereoscopic reels with the thought that the book will now be more accessible to both veterinary students and veterinary practitioners.

As is typical of surgical techniques, some of those presented in the first edition have been modified and clarified. Two new procedures, lobectomy and scrotal urethrostomy, which I felt would benefit the student as well as practicing veterinarians, have been added.

The new drawings have been done by George Batik. I wish to remind the readers that the original drawings were taken from three-dimensional photographs provided by Dr. Harlan Jensen.

I am again indebted to my wife, Willie, for her continued help with typing and everything else.

Richard E. Hoffer

Preface TO FIRST EDITION

The *Stereoscopic Atlas of Small Animal Surgery: Thoracic, Abdominal, and Soft Tissue Techniques* has been written to fill the need of veterinarians and veterinary students for a text that details each phase of the surgery. Through photography, artwork, and three-dimensional reels, Dr. Jensen and I hope to clarify the instructions for each surgical step. We feel the clearly shown anatomical relationships in the stereoscopic reels are of special value.

This is not intended to be a composite of all the surgery techniques, and we have not attempted to review or acknowledge the literature on soft tissue surgery. These are not original operations. Many of them have been used for years and are basic, standard procedures, but some of them have been modified to suit our needs. We present a workable and fundamental approach to each surgical problem and expect the individual surgeon to be inspired to modify them to suit his needs.

The methods and techniques are those that have proved successful for us. When more than one technique is described, the reader should select the one most applicable to his problem.

All the original drawings were done by Ronald Cherkas, biological artist and photographer. The stereo photography was done by Dr. Wayne Wingfield and Dr. Jensen with the Donaldson stereo camera.

I feel especially indebted to Dr. B. F. Hoerlein of Auburn University, Dr. L. E. Evans of Oklahoma State University, and Dr. R. L. Leighton of the University of California at Davis for their instruction and inspiration during my professional career. I am also grateful to many other colleagues who have read the manuscript and given constructive criticism prior to its publication.

I am indebted to my wife, Willie, for her help with the typing and to Naomi Jensen for her help in editing the text.

Richard E. Hoffer

Contents

PART ONE
GENERAL CONSIDERATIONS

1
Preoperative and postoperative care

Preoperative and postoperative care may make the difference between success and failure of the surgical procedure.

Preoperative care includes evaluation of the patient's physical and physiological status in relation to the anticipated surgery. It should also include the determination of any additional therapy the patient may need during the surgical procedure and the careful choice of the anesthetic agent.

Postoperative care begins when the incision is closed and continues until the patient is discharged. It includes treatment of any problems resulting from surgical manipulation, maintenance of the water, electrolyte, and nutritional balance by parenteral administration of fluids, and all therapy necessary to restore the patient to a normal physical and physiological status.

Although brief descriptions of some of the principles of preoperative and postoperative considerations are presented, the reader is referred to the references for more abundant information in the various areas.

PREOPERATIVE CARE

All patients should receive a thorough physical examination prior to surgery. The physical examination should include auscultation and palpation. Ideally all patients should be evaluated by clinical pathological data, including a complete blood count (CBC), blood urea nitrogen evaluation (BUN), urinalysis, and heartworm check. If the patient is over 5 years of age, a serum glutamic transaminase evaluation should also be done. These procedures give the surgeon a baseline on which to evaluate the patient's postoperative progress. Many times a good preoperative evaluation will uncover other conditions that may lead to reassessment of the advisability of surgery or that may influence the result of surgery, for example, congenital heart defects, early systemic disease, or heartworms.

Before surgery, patients should have a catheter placed in the cephalic or jugular vein to receive appropriate fluids during the surgical procedure. Fluids to be replaced include those lost during the preoperative fasting period, as well as those lost in the critical patient through vomitimg or diarrhea. Also, if it suddenly becomes necessary to administer blood or drugs during the surgical procedure, the intravenous catheter will have maintained an opening into the cardiovascular system.

The choice of anesthesia must be considered a part of the preoperative decision. All the procedures described in this atlas are performed with either methoxyflurane and oxygen or halothane and oxygen anesthesia. Generally the anesthesia is induced with a short-acting barbiturate after premedication with atropine. A cuffed endotracheal tube is placed in the trachea, and during the procedure the anesthesia is maintained with the gas mixture.

There are numerous methods of monitoring the blood pressure, heart rate, and urine output. The equipment necessary to do this varies in sophistication and may cost from a few dollars to thousands of dollars. Generally the monitoring of central venous pressure in addition to electrocardiogram (ECG) will give the surgeon much information at a relatively small cost. This type of monitoring is very important.

POSTOPERATIVE CARE

Postoperative care of the patient is one of the most important facets of surgery. This is especially true of the geriatric patient and the patient critically ill prior to surgical intervention.

The most important aspect of postoperative care is close observation of the patient. Standard parameters that should be observed are body temperature, urine output, capillary refill, respiratory rate and character, pulse rate and character, and heart sounds.

ECG monitoring and measurement of central venous pressure will add additional information that is especially important after thoracic surgery. The postoperative administration of fluids can be more closely regulated when central venous pressure is monitored.

The objective of immediate postoperative observation is to anticipate postoperative complications such as shock, pulmonary edema, cardiac arrhythmias, or renal shutdown and to prevent their occurrence. It is easier on the patient to prevent a complication than to administer emergency treatment in an attempt to reverse the complications. The more sophisticated the equipment the surgeon has available, the more parameters that can be monitored. However, even without sophisticated equipment, the percentage of post-surgical survival can be greatly increased by just closely observing the vital signs of the patient. Additional postoperative procedures such as aspiration of chest tubes or peritoneal lavage and dialysis will be dictated by the procedures performed.

The immediate postoperative period ends after the animal has recovered from the anesthetic and the vital signs have stabilized. The rest of the postoperative treatment will depend on the procedure performed, the animal's response to the surgery, and the condition that warranted the surgery.

This period of time is especially important in the geriatric patient. The surgeon should not forget that not only does the surgical problem have to be treated but also the patient has to be maintained in a good physical and physiological state in order to recover and heal. The possible loss of the older patient from such secondary factors as renal failure or congestive heart failure following the stress of surgery and subsequent hospitalization must be anticipated and prevented.

In summary, postoperative care of the patient includes the following:
1. Immediate treatment of postsurgical and anesthetic complications
2. Anticipation, prevention, or treatment of possible postsurgical problems resulting from the stress of surgery, the predisposing disease that required the surgery, or the animal's physiological response during the period of hospitalization

The above can be accomplished with a minimum amount of equipment but requires the time and interest of the surgeon.

REFERENCES

Brasmer, T. H.: Symposium on shock, Vet. Clin. North Am. 6:entire issue, 1976.

Finco, D. R., and Osborne, C. A.: Practical application of principles of fluid and electrolyte therapy. In Proceedings of the American Animal Hospital Association, Elkhart, Ind., 1972, The Association, p. 210.

Knowles, R. P.: Intensive care, J. Am. Anim. Hosp. Assoc. 8 (special issue), 1972.

Martin, D. B.: Applicable procedures for the intensive care patient. In Proceedings of the American Animal Hospital Association, Elkhart, Ind., 1972, The Association, p. 276.

Sattler, F. B.: The intensive care patient. In Proceedings of the American Animal Hospital Association, Elkhart, Ind., 1969, The Association, p. 281.

Soma, L. R., editor: Textbook of veterinary anesthesia, Baltimore, 1971, The Williams & Wilkins Co.

2
Aseptic surgery

The procedures presented in this atlas are performed utilizing standard aseptic surgical principles, which are discussed and well illustrated in many textbooks of surgery. Following is a brief review of the methods of preparation of the patient and surgeon for aseptic surgery.

PATIENT PREPARATION

The hair in the operative area is clipped with a fine surgical blade. It is good practice to clip at least twice the area thought to be necessary for performing the surgical procedure. In this way, if a larger incision is required to recover from a surgical emergency, it can be made without contaminating the surgical field. Preparation of a large area also eliminates the problem of contamination that could result if the surgical drapes should become displaced.

The area is scrubbed at least three times with a germicidal soap, and liberal quantities of water are used to rinse the site. The animal is carefully transported to the operating room, where an antiseptic is applied to the prepared surgical area.

PREPARATION OF THE SURGEON AND ASSISTANTS

Caps, masks, and hoods are donned before the operating room is entered. The linen packs are placed on a table and opened. The instrument pack is placed on a Mayo operating stand and partially opened. The wraps are spread appropriately to minimize contamination from the top of the instrument table.

After the surgeon first scrubs his hands and forearms with a germicidal soap, he cleans his fingernails. The final surgical scrub employs a brush or disposable soap-impregnated sponge. The basic rule to follow is to start with the fingers and fingernails, using twenty strokes of the brush on each surface of the fingers, hands, and forearms and twenty strokes on the fingernails. The hands are rinsed, allowing the water to run off the elbows, and are dried with a sterile towel.

After the surgeon has gowned, he puts on the gloves so that the un-

6

gloved hand touches only the inside of the glove. The gloves are smoothed over the hands, and the patient is draped.

The surgical site can be draped by a variety of methods. A four-quadrant draping method using 48-inch by 48-inch double-thickness muslin drapes may be used. The drapes are placed on the patient by folding the edge of the drape over the hand to prevent contamination of the gloves. The posterior drape continues up over the Mayo stand. The drapes are fixed to the patient at each corner of the anticipated incision site with towel clamps. Additional towel clamps are used where necessary to prevent sagging or gapping of the drapes. An additional shroud or adhesive plastic drape is frequently used.

REFERENCES

Knecht, C. D., Welser, J. R., Allen, A. R., Williams, D. J., and Harris, N. N.: Fundamental techniques in veterinary surgery, Philadelphia, 1975, W. B. Saunders Co.

Leonard, E. P.: Fundamentals of small animal surgery, Philadelphia, 1968, W. B. Saunders Co.

Richards, R. E.: Surgical skin preparation. In Proceedings of the American Animal Hospital Association, Elkhart, Ind., 1972, The Association, p. 630.

PART TWO
THORAX

3
Thoracic exposures and closure

Thoracotomy is the approach of choice for most thoracic surgery in the dog or cat. There are four basic thoracotomy incisions. The left cranial chest may be approached between the left fourth and fifth ribs. This approach is utilized for repair of a patent ductus arteriosus (Chapter 4) or other procedures involving the great thoracic vessels. An incision made between the left fifth and sixth ribs will expose more of the heart but still permits access to the great vessels. The right cranial chest is approached either between the right fourth and fifth or right fifth and sixth ribs. The cranial thoracic esophagus is best exposed by a right cranial thoracotomy (Chapter 5). The caudal chest is approached by a left or right thoracotomy between the eighth and ninth or ninth and tenth ribs. The thoracotomy approach for the modified Heller procedure (Chapter 6) is made in the left eighth or ninth thoracic interspace.

Esophagotomy may also be performed through a left caudal thoracotomy. However, if the surgeon anticipates the need for esophageal resection and anastomosis, a right caudal thoracotomy should be performed, since this permits better exposure and mobilization of the esophagus. In general, esophageal surgery is most effectively performed through a right thoracotomy. To remove esophageal foreign bodies, the surgeon should make the thoracotomy incision through the intercostal space closest to the foreign body. The location of the foreign body can be determined by radiography prior to surgery.

THORACIC EXPOSURES

The basic surgical techniques for various thoracotomy approaches are the same. Incisions are made through individual tissue layers. Since the field should be dry before the chest is entered, bleeding in each layer is controlled by ligation with 3-0 gut. The thoracotomy incision is made through the intercostal muscles midway between the two ribs. This will avoid the intercostal vessels caudal to the rib, as well as the ventral intercostal vessels cranial to the rib.

Plate 1. Cranial thoracic approach

A The skin *(1)*, subcutaneous tissue *(2)*, and cutaneous trunci muscle *(3)* are incised. The incision begins immediately caudal to the scapula. Bleeding is controlled by ligation with 3-0 gut. The subcutaneous tissue is incised until the latissimus dorsi muscle *(4)* is exposed. Bleeding should be completely controlled before the next layer is incised.

B The ventral border of the latissimus dorsi muscle *(1)* is identified, and scissors *(2)* are slipped under it to identify the tissue plane. The latissimus dorsi muscle is incised. Again all bleeders are controlled before proceeding to the next layer. At this point the surgeon may slip his finger under the latissimus dorsi and palpate the first rib. By counting back, the exact intercostal space can be determined.

C The latissimus dorsi muscle *(1)* has been incised, exposing the serratus ventralis thoracalis *(2)* and the external abdominal oblique *(3)*. The muscles are separated in the direction of their fibers to expose the underlying external intercostal muscles. Bleeding is controlled before proceeding.

D The serratus *(1)* is being reflected with an Allis tissue forceps. The external and internal intercostal muscles *(2)* have been incised simultaneously, exposing the pleura *(3)*. The intercostal muscles are initially opened with scissors down to the pleura. The scissors are placed with one blade in the tissue plane between the pleura and internal intercostal and the other blade outside the external intercostal muscle. The muscles are then carefully cut, preserving the pleura. If the surgeon desires, the intercostal muscle and pleura may be incised as a block, with care being taken not to damage the lungs.

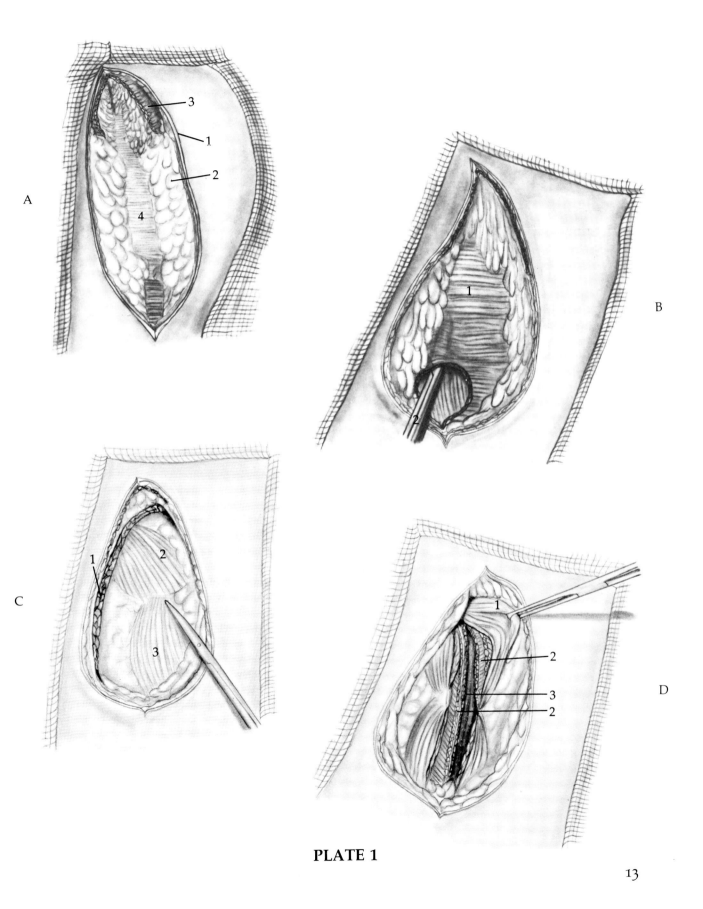

PLATE 1

13

Plate 2. Cranial thoracic approach

A   The pleura has been incised, and the ribs spread with a rib spreader. A small stab incision was made through the pleura, and this incision was enlarged with a scissors. The cranial *(1)* and middle *(2)* lobes of the left lung are seen, as well as the aorta *(3)*, the brachiocephalic artery *(4)*, the left subclavian artery *(5)*, and the left pulmonary artery *(6)*. The lungs obscure the rest of the field, but a small portion of the heart *(7)* may be seen.

B   The lungs have been reflected caudally, exposing the thoracic viscera. The aorta *(1)*, pulmonary artery *(2)*, left subclavian artery *(3)*, and heart *(4)* are clearly seen. The vagus *(5)* and phrenic *(6)* nerves are seen. Note the difference between this illustration and the illustration of the cranial thoracic approach used for a patent ductus arteriosus (Chapter 4). The thymus gland *(7)* is seen cranial to the heart in young dogs.

C   The right cranial thorax has been exposed. The cranial *(1)* and middle *(2)* lobes of the lung have been reflected caudally, and the cranial vena cava *(3)* and vagus nerve *(4)* are visualized. The esophagus is located in the dorsal aspect of the cranial mediastinum *(5)*, along with the trachea. The incision is in the fifth intercostal space. Better esophageal exposure could be obtained by a thoracotomy through the fourth space.

More details of the cranial and caudal chest are presented in the chapters dealing with specific thoracic surgical procedures.

14

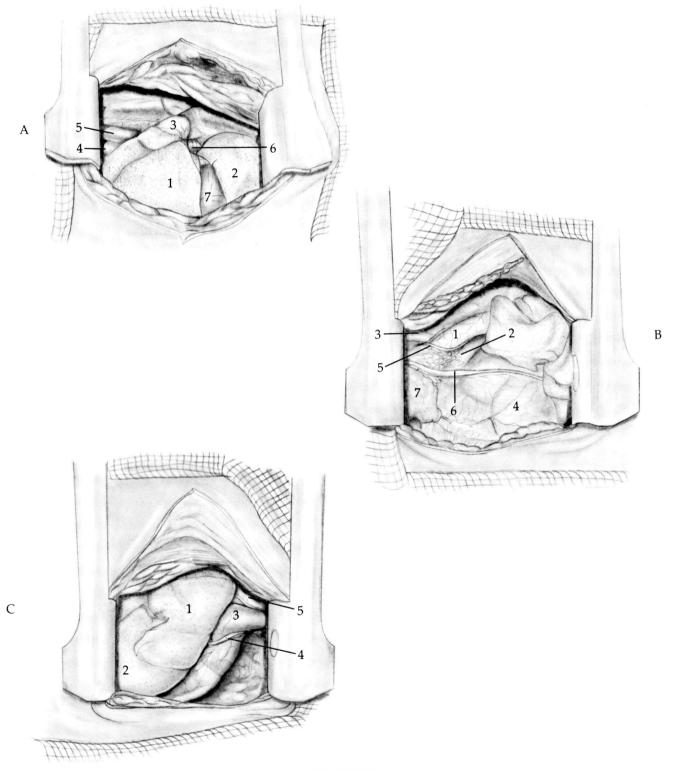

PLATE 2

Plate 3. Caudal thoracic approach

The skin incision for caudal thoracotomy should be made from the ventral extent of the epaxial muscles to a point below the costochondral junction.

A An incision through the skin *(1)*, subcutaneous tissue, cutaneous trunci, and latissimus dorsi *(2)* has been made between the eighth *(3)* and ninth *(4)* ribs. This exposes the external abdominal oblique muscle *(5)*. All bleeding has been controlled. The scissors *(6)* are slipped between the external abdominal oblique and the external intercostal muscles *(7)*, and the external abdominal oblique muscle is severed.

B The external abdominal oblique muscle *(1)* and the latissimus dorsi *(2)* have been incised, exposing the external intercostal muscle *(3)*. At this point the surgeon should check the intercostal space by sliding his fingers under the latissimus dorsi toward the last rib and counting the intercostal spaces. Remember there are twelve intercostal spaces and thirteen ribs. Incision of the external intercostal muscle has been started. The intercostal muscles and pleura may be incised as a unit, or the muscles may be incised separately from the pleura. With the latter approach there is less chance of lung damage. When the chest is to be entered, the lungs should be collapsed so that they are not damaged by the incision. Positive-pressure ventilation should be stopped while entry is being accomplished.

C The left chest has been entered, and the ribs spread with a rib spreader *(1)*. The caudal lobe *(2)* and a portion of the middle lobe *(3)* of the left lung are seen. The diaphragm *(4)* is also visualized.

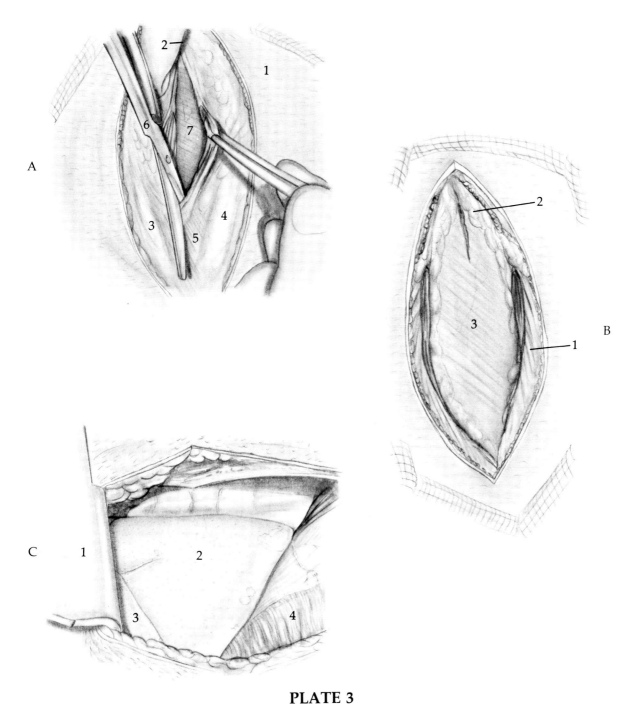

PLATE 3

Plate 4. Caudal thoracic approach

A The pulmonary ligament has been severed and the lung lobe reflected cranially, exposing the posterior left thoracic cavity. An Allis tissue forceps *(1)* is reflecting the diaphragm caudally and laterally. This exposes the phrenoesophageal ligament *(2)* as it reflects from the diaphragm *(3)* to the esophagus *(4)*. The dorsal *(5)* and ventral *(6)* vagal trunks are seen on the esophagus in the mediastinum. The aorta *(7)* is seen dorsal to the esophagus, and the phrenic nerve *(8)* is also visualized.

B The right caudal chest has been exposed. The caudal lobe *(1)* of the lung is in traction, exposing the pulmonary ligament *(2)*. This ligament must be incised to reflect the lung cranially. The accessory lobe *(3)* of the lung lies over the esophagus. The caudal vena cava *(4)* and phrenic nerve *(5)* may be seen approaching the diaphragm *(6)*. A portion of the middle lobe *(7)* of the lung is also visualized.

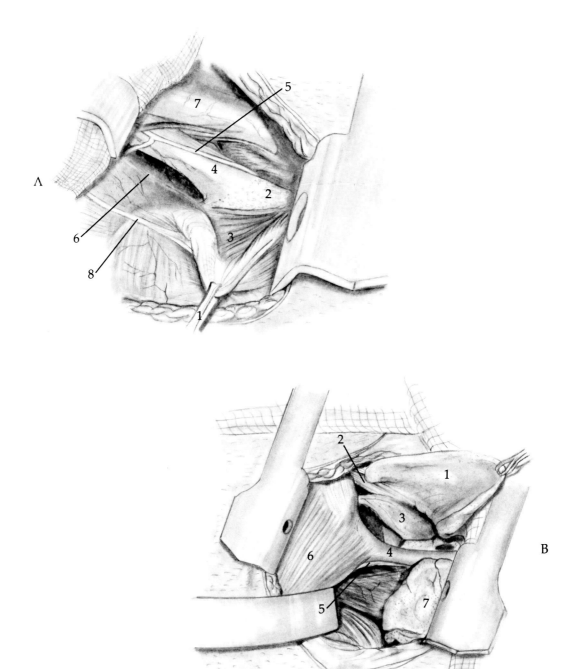

PLATE 4

THORACIC CLOSURE

The basic technique for closing a thoracotomy is the same for all sites of incision. The closure is sutured layer by layer, as the thorax was opened.

Before a thoracotomy is closed, a chest tube should be placed. The diameter of the tube will vary according to the size of the patient. Silastic medical-grade tubing, which is nonreactive, pliable, and yet firm enough not to collapse, may be used. A trocar type chest tube of polyvinyl chloride may also be used. This is easier to place and comes prepackaged. The tube should be firm enough to remain patent but soft enough not to damage the thoracic viscera.

The ventral mediastinum is severed so that both sides of the chest communicate freely before the tube is placed. This will prevent the pocketing of air or fluid on the side of the chest away from the tube. The lung should be fully expanded before closing the chest.

Plate 5. Thoracic closure

A A small incision has been made 6 cm from the thoracotomy incision. The incision goes through the skin and subcutaneous tissue. A Carmalt forceps (1) is placed in the skin incision and forced through the subcutaneous tissue to the intercostal space behind the incision and then forced through the intercostal space so that it can grasp the chest tube. Note that the forceps is not visible except inside the chest (2). If the subcutaneous tissue over the area where the forceps penetrates the chest is broken and if the forceps is exposed before it enters the chest, the area will leak air, since the subcutaneous tissue seals the area where the forceps penetrates the muscles.

B The Carmalt forceps, along with the tube, has been withdrawn from the chest, and the chest tube is now in position. Generally it is preferable to have the chest tube in the ventral aspect of the thorax; however, this is not necessary. Multiple holes are cut in the chest tube (1) before placement. If the tube is placed high in the thorax, air is withdrawn by positioning the dog with the tube side up, and fluid is withdrawn by positioning the dog with the tube side down.

C Four to six Ethiflex* sutures are placed around the ribs, penetrating only the pleura and intercostal muscles. The sutures are passed by inserting a curved hemostat (1) with the suture (2) through the rib space cranial to the incision and grasping the suture with a second hemostat (3) placed through the intercostal space caudal to the incision. The use of a small hemostat should prevent damage to the intercostal arteries. If an intercostal artery should be damaged, bleeding can be controlled by passing two gut sutures about the rib, above and below the site of the bleeding.

D The first suture (1) is placed at the costochondral junction, the second (2) below it, and the last two to four are evenly spaced between the costochondral junction and the top of the incision. Care is taken not to include the chest tube in any of the sutures.

After all the sutures have been placed, the ribs are apposed, and the sutures are tied. The ribs should be in exact apposition; they should not overlap.

Heavy surgical gut may be utilized for rib sutures in smaller dogs. In large dogs, No. 1 Ethiflex makes an excellent rib suture.

---

*Ethicon Co., Somerville, N.J.

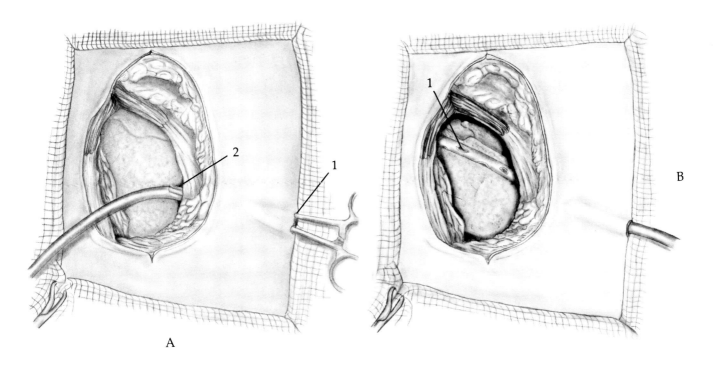

A

B

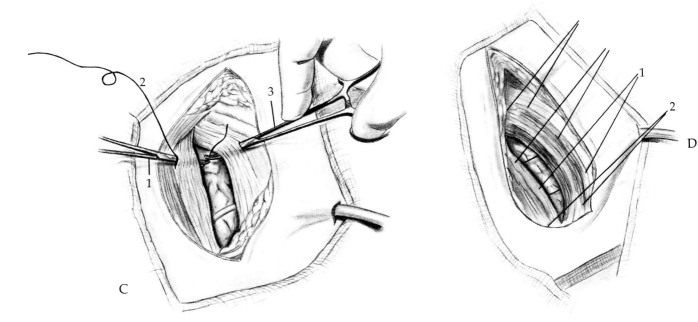

C

D

PLATE 5

21

Plate 6. Thoracic closure

A The intercostal muscles and fascia are closed with a simple continuous suture pattern *(1)* using surgical gut. The serratus ventralis thoracalis *(2)* and the external abdominal oblique muscles *(3)* are closed with simple interrupted sutures of absorbable material. A simple interrupted suture *(4)* is being placed in the latissimus dorsi muscle.

B The latissimus dorsi *(1)* has been completely closed with simple interrupted sutures, and the subcutaneous tissue *(2)* is being closed with simple interrupted sutures of absorbable material.

C The skin is closed with simple interrupted sutures of nonabsorbable material. The chest tube *(1)* has been fixed to the skin by a mattress suture *(2)*. The ends of the mattress suture are left long enough to tie the tube to the skin *(3)* with this suture. Care is taken not to penetrate the tube with the mattress suture.

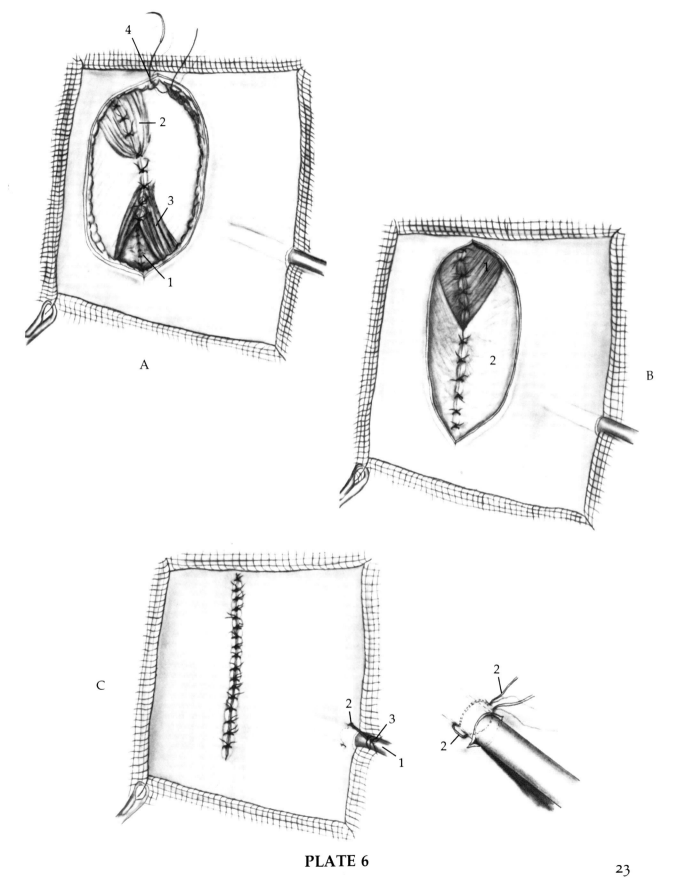

A

B

C

PLATE 6

23

POSTOPERATIVE CARE

The chest tube is aspirated following closure of the chest to establish a negative pressure. After surgery the tube is aspirated every hour until less than 2 cc per hour of fluid or air is obtained for 2 successive hours. The tube may then be aspirated 8 hours later. If there is less than 10 cc of air or fluid after 8 to 10 hours, the tube may be removed. If more fluid is present, the tube is left until a total of only 1 cc per hour is removed.

To maintain negative pressure the tube may be occluded by a three-way stopcock, but if this is not available, a Carmalt forceps may be used. A Heimlich valve (see Appendix) may also be used. This is best utilized for removing air but will allow the escape of fluid. However, if there is a lot of blood, the valve may become occluded and not function properly. The surgeon should remember that a dog with a chest tube, regardless of the method of occlusion, should be closely observed. The tube, clamp, or valve is taped to the dog's chest or abdomen to prevent inadvertent pulling of the tube.

To remove the chest tube a mattress suture is placed through the skin and around the tube. The suture is partially tied, and tension is put on it while the tube is pulled out of the chest. The suture is then tied, closing the defect created by the tube.

A caudal thoracotomy involves different muscles but is closed in the same manner. The rib sutures are first placed and tied. The intercostal muscles are sutured with a simple continuous suture, and the external abdominal oblique and latissimus dorsi muscles are closed with simple interrupted sutures. Placement of the chest tube is identical to that in a cranial thoracotomy.

Antibiotics should be used after placement of a chest tube to reduce the incidence of ascending infection. Chest drains, as is true of all drains, should be left in position only as long as necessary.

REFERENCE

Sauer, B. W.: Valve drainage of the pleural cavity of the dog, J. Am. Vet. Med. Assoc. **155**:1997, 1969.

4
Patent ductus arteriosus repair

Two techniques for repairing a patent ductus arteriosus will be described. The method of ligation is the simplest technique, requiring the least amount of equipment and time, whereas division of the ductus followed by suture of the pulmonic and aortic sides of the ductus requires more equipment, skill, and time.

The ligation method of repair may be used only when the ductus is longer than it is wide. If ligation is attempted on a short, wide ductus, the suture may cut through the ductus, resulting in massive hemorrhage.

Division of the ductus with suture repair of the two cut ends may be utilized to repair any type of patent ductus arteriosus, whether long or short. It should be used when there is any indication that the ligation method will sever the ductus.

The basic exposure and handling of the aorta and pulmonary arteries are the same for both procedures. The placement of umbilical tapes around the aorta prior to manipulation of the ductus gives the surgeon complete control of aortic bleeding. If the aorta or ductus is damaged, the tapes can be tightened, allowing time for the surgeon to obtain control of the defect without major blood loss.

Plate 7. Patent ductus arteriosus

A A left fourth intercostal thoracotomy has been performed (Chapter 3). The cranial portion of the left atrium *(1)*, the aorta *(2)*, the pulmonary artery *(3)*, and the ductus arteriosus *(4)* are exposed. These are covered by the transparent intact pericardial sac and pericardial mediastinum. The left vagus nerve *(5)* and left phrenic nerve *(6)* are located in these tissues as they pass over the ductus. The pulmonary artery and aorta may show a dilatation at the point of entry of the ductus. Because this area is thin and more friable than the remainder of the vessels, it is easily damaged. A dilatation of the pulmonary outflow tract is usually seen and appears much thinner than the rest of the pulmonary artery. The ductus arteriosus is located caudal to the left subclavian artery and cranial to the bifurcation of the main pulmonary artery.

B The pericardial sac has been incised between the left vagus nerve *(1)* and the phrenic nerve *(2)*. Stay sutures of 0 silk *(3)* have been passed around the nerves, and the cut edges of the pericardial sac and the nerves have been reflected dorsally and ventrally. In the smaller dog it may be easier to incise below the phrenic nerve and reflect the vagus nerve and the phrenic nerve dorsally. The connective tissue has been dissected free from the lateral aspect of the aorta and pulmonary artery. The connective tissue on the dorsal aspect of the aorta has been dissected free for a short distance on either side of the entry of the ductus arteriosus. The connective tissue between the aorta and pulmonary artery, cranial and caudal to the ductus arteriosus, has been freed by blunt-scissor dissection. The hemostat *(4)* is holding an umbilical tape prior to passing it around the aorta.

C A right-angle Mixter forceps *(1)* has been passed dorsal and medial to the aorta so that the point emerges cranial to the ductus arteriosus. An 18-inch (¼ inch in diameter) umbilical tape *(2)* that has been soaked in saline is grasped by the forceps and pulled around the aorta. The umbilical tape is then passed through a boot (Appendix), clamped, and placed out of the field.

D Caudal to the ductus arteriosus, a second tape has been passed in the same manner as in Plate 7, C. When the forceps are being passed medial to the aorta, care must be taken and only slight pressure used in order not to perforate either the aorta or the pulmonary artery. Passage of the forceps may be facilitated by gently opening and closing the points so as to separate the connective tissue. The forceps are never forced, and gentle traction at the separation of the pulmonary artery and aorta will aid in exposing the point of the forceps.

After the umbilical tapes are in place, the surgeon has better control of the aorta. If the ductus should be inadvertently injured, aortic hemorrhage may be controlled by tightening both boots and repairing the defect. Pulmonary arterial hemorrhage may be controlled by digital pressure until a vascular clamp may be applied.

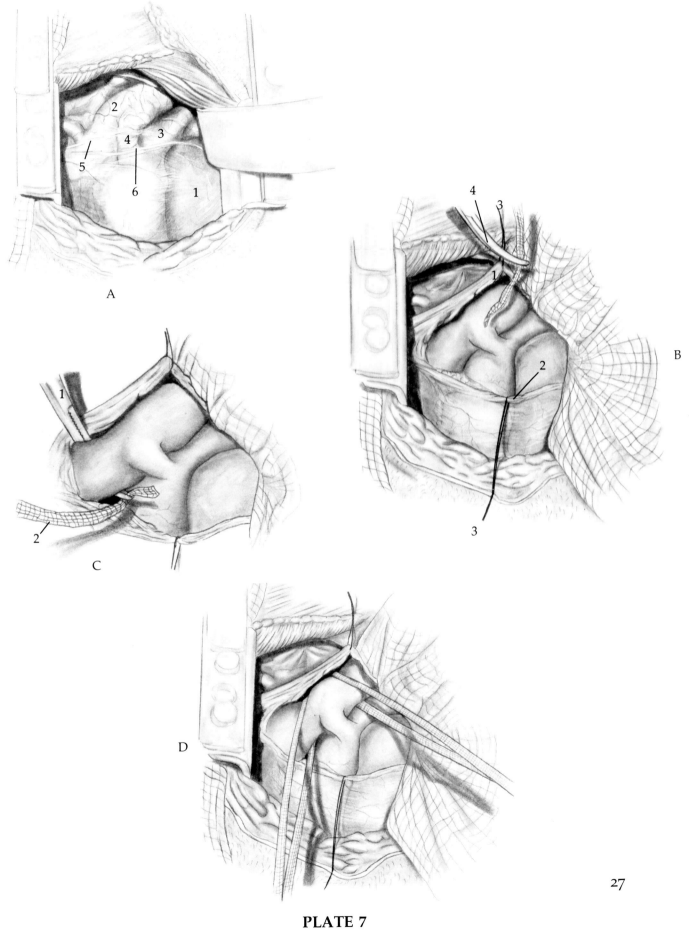

A

B

C

D

27

PLATE 7

Plate 8. Patent ductus arteriosus

A The cranial and caudal aspects of the ductus arteriosus and the areas on the aorta and pulmonary artery where the ductus enters have been carefully cleaned of connective tissue. The ductus, aorta, and pulmonary artery may be gently grasped with a Potts thumb forceps and manipulated to facilitate the dissection. Connective tissue must be removed before the vessels can be sutured or clamped. If the connective tissue is not removed, it may interfere with closure of the ductus or obscure the surgical site. The medial aspect of the ductus has been cleaned by putting gentle traction on the umbilical tapes in a lateral ventral direction. This will roll the aorta away from the vertebrae, exposing the medial aspect of the ductus arteriosus and pulmonary artery. These structures can then be cleaned of connective tissue under direct visualization. The aorta should not be completely occluded while it is being elevated.

B A right-angle forceps (3) has been passed medial to the ductus arteriosus. The passage of the forceps may be facilitated and the aortic and pulmonic arterial dilatation guarded by rolling the aorta laterally and ventrally. This allows the forceps to be passed under direct visualization and decreases the possibility of puncturing these structures. A 0 silk ligature (1) has been passed medial to the ductus arteriosus. Gentle traction is placed on the first ligature, and the right-angle forceps is again passed medial to the ductus arteriosus. A second 0 silk ligature (2) is grasped by the right-angle forceps (3). The forceps are withdrawn, resulting in two ligatures being placed medial to the ductus arteriosus. If the surgeon prefers, umbilical tape, which is less likely to sever the ductus, may be used instead of silk for ligation.

C Gentle traction is placed on the lower ligature (1) while the upper ligature (2) is tied. Then the traction is reversed, and the lower ligature is tied. By careful traction, the ligatures may be placed close to the aorta and pulmonary artery.

D Note that both ligatures have been tied and that there is some distance between them. This is obtained by careful traction while tying the sutures. Care must be taken when applying traction not to tear the aortic or pulmonic attachment of the ductus arteriosus. The ligatures must be tightened slowly. If they appear as if they will cut through the ductus arteriosus or result in tearing of the ductus arteriosus, the ligatures are not tightened and the division and suture method of repair is used.

It is best to temporarily occlude the ductus before tying the sutures to evaluate the effect on cardiac function. This is especially important if there is increased right ventricular pressure.

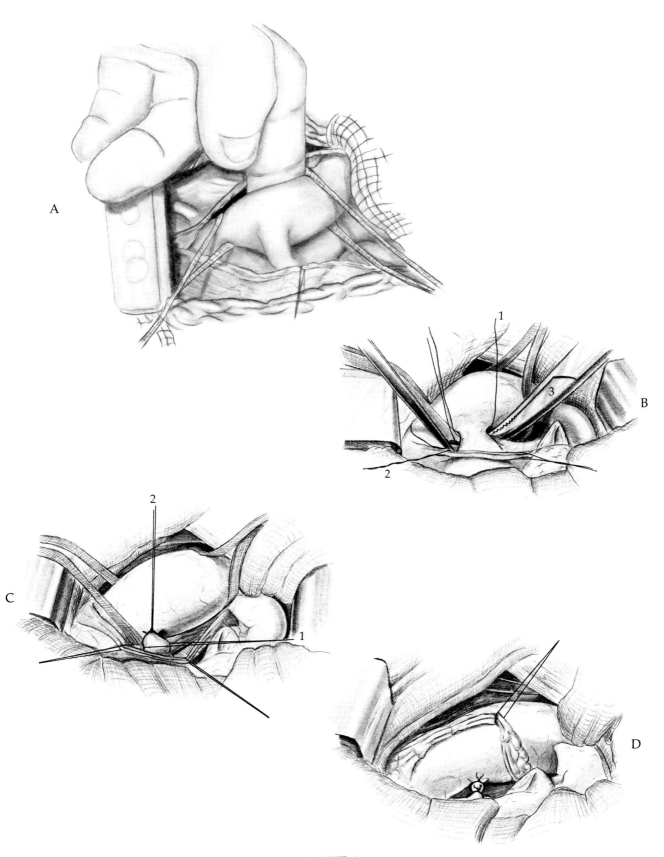

PLATE 8

Plate 9. Patent ductus arteriosus

A To use the division and suture method, the ductus is exposed as described in plates 7, *A*, through 8, *A*. After the ductus and its entry into the aorta and pulmonary artery have been dissected free of connective tissue, a Cooley pediatric vessel forceps *(1)* (see Appendix) is placed across the aortic side of the ductus arteriosus, including a portion of the aorta *(2)*. The length and configuration of the ductus arteriosus dictate the type of clamps used. If the duct is short, it is necessary to include a portion of the aorta or the pulmonary artery, or both, in the clamp. This will, in effect, make the ductus longer, since the clamp does not impinge on the ductus. Since it is more easily applied to the aorta, the Cooley forceps exposes more ductus than the straight patent ductus forceps. Care must be taken when passing the forceps because a sawing action of the jaws could result in a perforation of the ductus arteriosus or the aorta. The passage of the forceps may be faciltated by rolling the aorta as described in Plate 8, *B*. The forceps should be closed slowly to allow the circulatory system to adjust to the changes in blood flow and pressure and to evaluate the patient's response to occlusion.

B A second Cooley pediatric vessel forceps *(1)* is placed across the ductus arteriosus *(2)*, including a portion of the pulmonary artery *(3)*. Care must be taken in passing this forceps not to damage the pulmonary artery by any sawing or tearing action. Once both forceps are in position, they are held by the assistant, preventing a sharp pull or sawing action that would tear the ductus arteriosus, pulmonary artery, or aorta, while the surgeon is dividing the ductus.

C The ductus arteriosus has been divided midway between the two forceps with a scalpel. Care must be taken not to cut the ductus on a bias. The forceps are rotated so that the cut ends of the ductus arteriosus are facing the surgeon. This is done gently to prevent tearing of the great vessels.

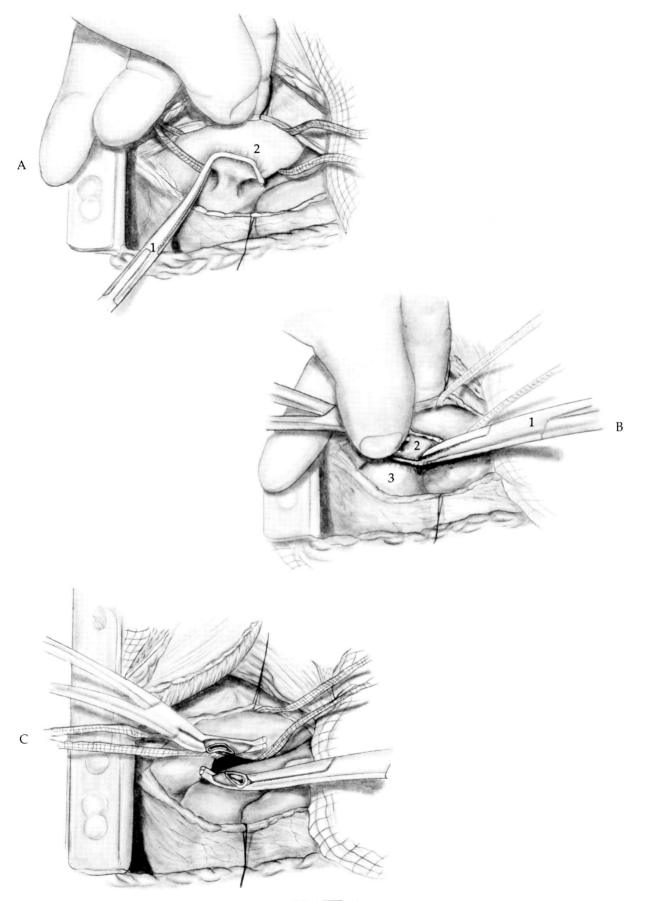

PLATE 9

Plate 10. Patent ductus arteriosus

A   The aorta and pulmonary artery are closed with a two-row crisscrossing continuous suture of 5-0 cardiovascular silk with a swaged needle. The aortic side of the ductus is sutured first *(1)*. The initial stitch is placed at one end of the ductus and tied; the loose end *(2)* is left long. The suture that is carried to the end of the incision *(3)* should be kept taut by gentle traction. If even tension is not maintained, the suture line will leak. If too much tension is applied, the suture will tear out. The suture pattern is reversed when the end is reached. The needle is placed at the same level but in between the first row of stitches *(4)*. As this row is tightened, it produces a crisscross effect *(5)* and seals the vessel without decreasing the lumen. The second row is carried to the end where the first row was started and is tied to the loose end *(6)*. The areas of closure most likely to leak are at the ends of the incision. The suture placement is critical at these points. The aortic forceps is slowly released to allow some blood to reach the suture line, then is reclamped for 7 minutes to allow the suture line to seal with fibrin. At the end of 7 minutes the forceps is removed completely and the suture line is examined for excessive bleeding. A small amount of suture-line bleeding is expected and can usually be controlled by applying pressure with a sponge. If there is any major spurting of blood, a simple interrupted suture of 5-0 silk is used to close the defect. After suturing has been completed, time must be allowed for these sutures to seal.

B   The pulmonic side of the ductus arteriosus is repaired in exactly the same way as described for the aortic side. The chest is cleaned of blood by suction and then lavaged with 500 ml of sterile saline solution. Aqueous penicillin at the dosage of 20,000 units per pound of body weight may be instilled in the chest prior to closure. The aortic and pulmonic suture lines are examined for bleeding; if the suture lines are dry, the umbilical tapes are cut close to the aorta and removed, and the stay sutures are removed from the pericardium. Then the pericardium is closed loosely with three to four simple interrupted sutures of chromic gut.

The mediastinum is perforated ventral to the heart to allow free drainage from both sides of the chest, a chest tube is placed, and the chest is closed (Chapter 3). After surgery the patient is closely observed until recovered from the anesthesia. The chest tube is usually removed 24 hours after surgery.

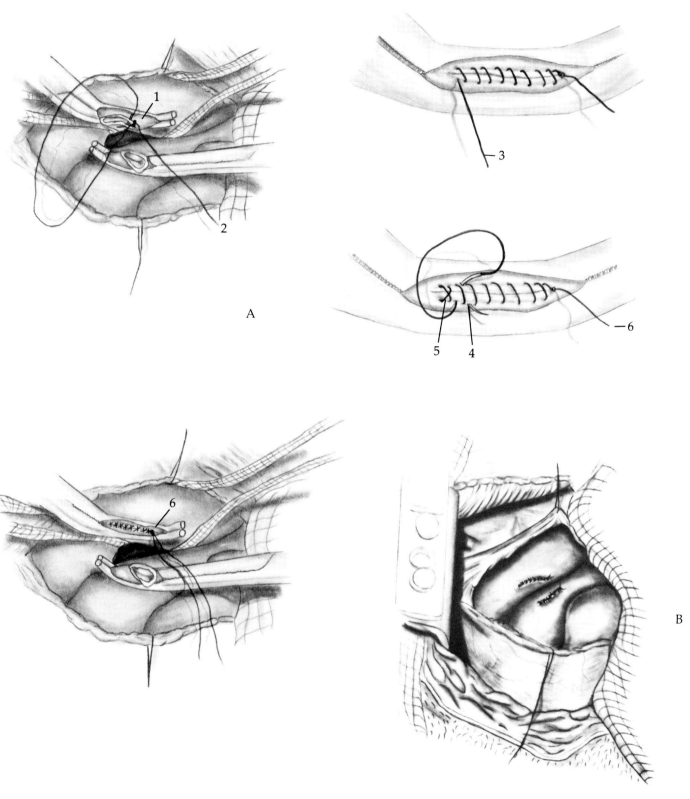

A

B

PLATE 10

REFERENCES

Buchanan, J. W.: Surgical treatment of congenital cardiovascular diseases. In Kirk, R. W., editor: Current veterinary therapy, 1966-1967, Philadelphia, 1966, W. B. Saunders Co.

Buchanan, J. W.: Symposium: thoracic surgery in the dog and cat. III. Patent ductus arteriosus and persistent right aortic arch surgery in dogs, J. Small Anim. Pract. **9**:409, 1968.

Patterson, D. F.: Diagnosis of congenital heart disease in small animal practice. In Proceedings of the American Animal Hospital Association, Elkhart, Ind., 1968, The Association, p. 27.

5
Esophagotomy

An esophagotomy is performed to remove a foreign object from the esophagus. A gastroscope may be used to examine or to attempt to remove the object. However, if the foreign body will not easily dislodge, and/or the operator has not had experience with the equipment, it is preferable to perform an esophagotomy rather than risk perforating or devitalizing esophageal tissue.

The location of the object determines the approach to be used. If the object is lodged in the cervical esophagus, a ventral midline cervical approach may be used. If the object is lodged in the esophagus cranial to the heart, a right thoracotomy should be used. If the object is lodged caudal to the heart, either a right or left thoracotomy may be used. If the surgeon anticipates having to resect the esophagus, a right thoracotomy is the approach of choice.

The esophagus does not have a serosal layer. Therefore the mucosal apposition is extremely important. The mucosal closure must be watertight when completed, since this provides the primary seal. The basic suture pattern to be described may be used for all esophageal surgery. However, if a resection and anastomosis is done, a simple interrupted suture pattern should be placed in the mucosa.

The esophagus is approached and the area evaluated. If the foreign body has been present long enough to produce an inflammatory response or if the object has perforated the esophagus, other tissues (such as the lung) may have adhered to the surgical site. Adhesions are carefully separated so as not to damage other structures such as the cranial vena cava or aorta. This potential problem can be eliminated by clearly visualizing the esophagus and structures close to it that the foreign body can damage if improperly manipulated.

Plate 11. Esophagotomy

A A right fourth thoracotomy has been performed (Chapter 3). The lung adhesions have been taken down and the lungs *(1)* packed out of the operative site. A fishhook *(2)* can be seen penetrating the esophagus *(3)*. Note the proximity of the aorta *(4)* and cranial vena cava *(5)*. The cranial mediastinum *(6)* has been carefully dissected from the esophagus, with care taken to preserve the nerves located in the mediastinum *(7)*. Branches of the vagus nerves to the esophagus, lungs, and heart are all located in the mediastinum in this area. The vagal trunks are located in the mediastinum over the esophagus (Chapter 3). These nerves within the mediastinum should be reflected when the esophagus is exposed.

B The esophagus is elevated from the mediastinum by bluntly stripping the mediastinum off the esophagus with scissors and digital manipulation, taking caution to preserve all nerves. While manipulating the esophagus, the surgeon should be careful that foreign bodies do not damage the major vessels in the area. Intestinal clamps *(1)* are applied cranial and caudal to the foreign body, including viable tissue. The esophagus may then be packed off within the limits of the space available. The fishhook has been grasped with a hemostat to prevent its damaging other structures. The esophagus is incised where the hook emerges *(2)*. If the foreign body is a sharp bone, the incision is made in tissue that has not been devitalized by pressure from the foreign body.

If there is a small necrotic area, this may be excised at this time. The decision to excise the necrotic area or resect the segment of esophagus depends on the amount of tissue that has been devitalized. If excision will compromise the lumen of the esophagus or if an entire portion of the esophagus has been devitalized, the esophagus must be resected. The prognosis for resection and anastomosis of the thoracic esophagus is generally poor; consequently this decision must not be made lightly. Generally, performing an esophagotomy before there has been excessive manipulation will decrease the need for esophageal resection and anastomosis.

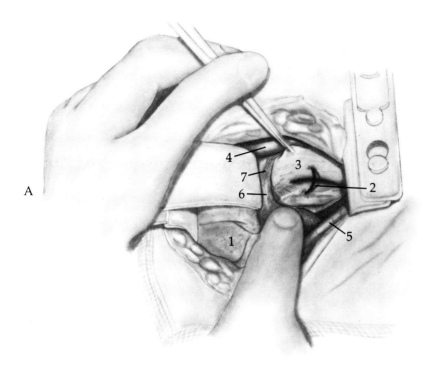

A

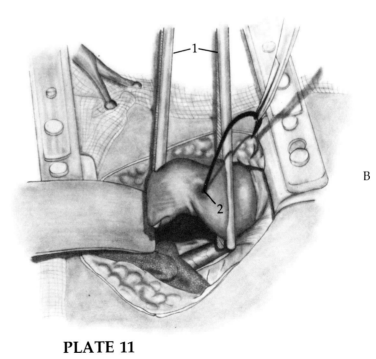

B

PLATE 11

Plate 12.   Esophagotomy

A   The esophagus has been incised. Note that the incision in the muscularis *(1)* extends cranial and caudal to the mucosal incision *(2)*.

B   A simple continuous suture of 5-0 silk with a swaged atraumatic needle is started at one corner of the mucosal incision *(1)*. This suture penetrates the submucosa and mucosa *(2)*.

C   The suture is carried to the opposite end of the mucosal incision and tied *(1)*. It is important that even tension be maintained on the suture line. This will prevent the first sutures from becoming loose while the final sutures are being placed. The closure of the mucosal incision is checked by injecting sterile saline solution into the esophageal lumen and applying pressure. Any leaks are closed with a simple interrupted suture of 5-0 silk in the mucosa and submucosa.

D   The muscularis is closed with a series of simple interrupted sutures of 3-0 chromic gut. This second suture line completely covers both ends of the mucosal incision *(1)*.

The esophagus should be rinsed with sterile saline solution before being returned to the chest. All instruments used for the esophagotomy are discarded. The operating stand and patient are redraped, and the surgeon changes gloves.

The chest is lavaged with 500 to 1000 ml of warm saline solution. A second lavage is done with a solution of 10 ml povidone-iodine (Betadine Whirlpool Concentrate*) in 1000 ml saline. The ventral mediastinum is broken down, a chest tube is placed, and the thorax is closed (Chapter 3).

Postoperatively the dog is maintained on parenteral fluids for 48 hours. Oral fluids are begun after 48 hours and continued until the fourth postoperative day, at which time a gruel may be fed. The dog should not receive solid food until at least the seventh postoperative day.

---

*Purdue Frederick Co., Norwalk, Conn.

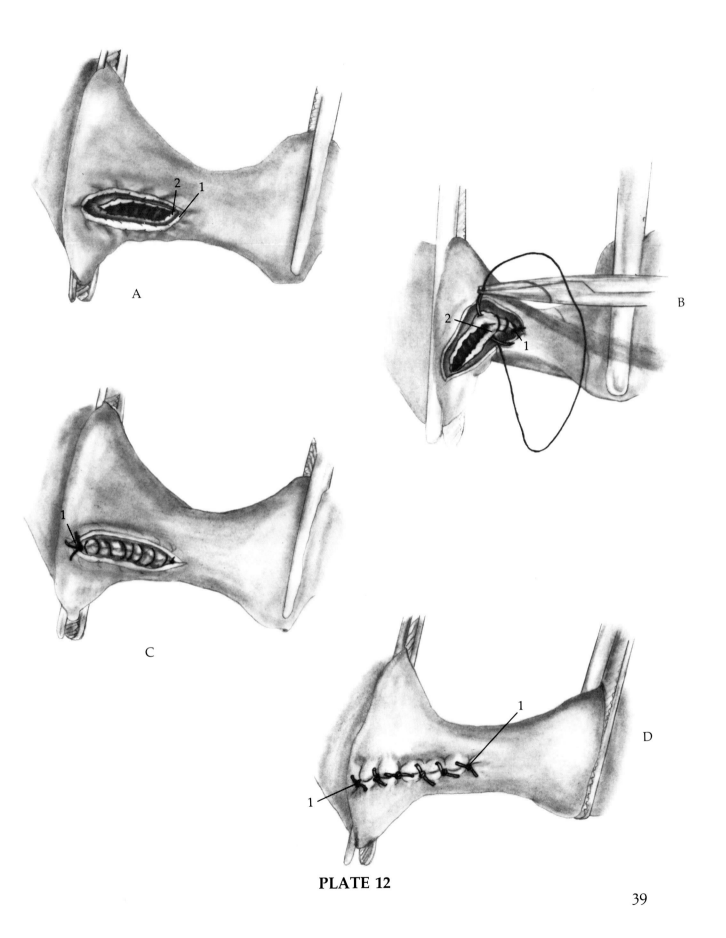

PLATE 12

REFERENCE

Ryan, W. W., and Greene, R. W.: The conservative management of esophageal foreign bodies and their complications: a review of 66 cases in dogs and cats, J.A.A.H.A. **11**:2043, 1975.

6
Modified Heller procedure

The modified Heller procedure, or esophagomyotomy, is performed for acquired achalasia. The operation severs the musculature at the gastroesophageal junction, the purpose of this being to relieve the functional obstruction produced by the failure of the cardia to relax synchronously when swallowing occurs.

The thoracotomy is performed through the left eighth and ninth rib space (Chapter 3).

Plate 13. Modified Heller procedure

A   The thorax has been entered. The pulmonary ligament has been severed, and the diaphragmatic lobe of the lung has been packed into the cranial thorax by use of a moist towel. The esophagus *(1)*, along with the dorsal *(2)* and ventral *(3)* vagal trunks in the mediastinum, is exposed. The aorta *(4)* can be seen dorsal to the esophagus. The phrenoesophageal ligament *(5)* is formed by the reflection of the diaphragmatic pleura and diaphragmatic peritoneum onto the esophagus. The diaphragm *(6)* is joined to the esophagus by this ligament. The diaphragm *(7)* has been retracted to expose this area.

B   The mediastinum will be incised and carefully reflected off the esophagus. The vagal trunks are reflected with the mediastinum; care must be taken not to damage them. A 1/4-inch latex tube *(1)* has been passed under the esophagus, and cranial traction is being applied to it. The diaphragm is being retracted caudally, thus stretching the phrenoesophageal ligament. The dorsolateral pleural portion of the phrenoesophageal ligament *(2)* has been incised. This incision will be lengthened, and the abdominal portion *(3)* of the phrenoesophageal ligament incised. Note the junction of the phrenoesophageal ligament and diaphragm *(4)*.

C   The incision through the phrenoesophageal ligament has been completed, exposing the cardia of the stomach *(1)*. Note the free border of the phrenoesophageal ligament *(2)* and the diaphragmatic edge *(3)*. Sutures *(4,5)* have been placed in the diaphragm and the free edge of the phrenoesophageal ligament. Note that the phrenoesophageal ligament incision is carried to the junction of the diaphragm with the muscularis of the esophagus *(6)*.

D   The surgeon's fingers are placed beneath the esophagus, and the esophagus is put on stretch. The muscular coat of the esophagus is incised down to the submucosa. This initial incision, which is made cranial to the cardia of the stomach, has to be done carefully because the esophageal mucosa must not be penetrated. Bleeding from the submucosa and from the muscular layer of the esophagus should be controlled by digital pressure. If there is a large muscular bleeder, it may be ligated. However, bleeders in the submucosa should not be ligated, since ligation of these could devitalize the tissue and result in a mucosal perforation.

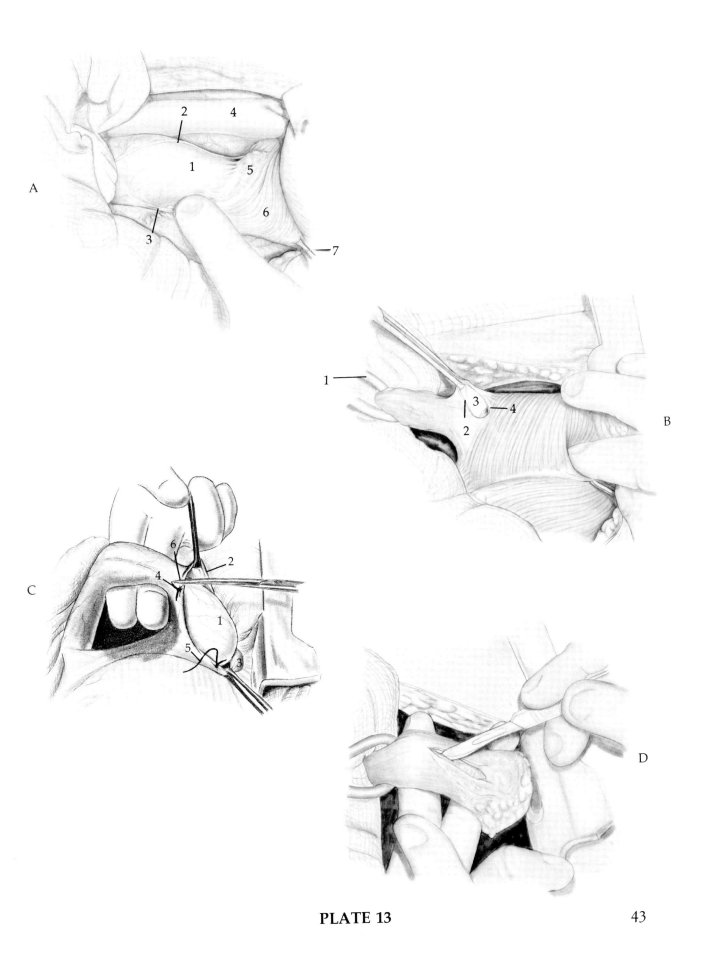

PLATE 13

Plate 14.   Modified Heller procedure

A   After the initial muscle incision has been made, a mosquito forceps is utilized to separate the helical muscle layers from the submucosa *(1)*. The closed forceps is passed gently between the two layers and opened. The muscle is then cut with a scissors. The delineation of the muscle layer from the submucosa is definite on the esophagus. This division becomes less pronounced as the gastroesophageal junction is approached.

B   The esophageal muscle incision is carried onto the cardia of the stomach. Since the muscular junction between the cardia and esophagus is not clearly defined, care should be taken when incising this area. A mosquito forceps is used to separate the musculature from the submucosa. Note the forceps under the circular layer of muscle at the cardia *(1)*. After incision of the muscles, the separation is enlarged by bluntly reflecting the edges of the muscle incision with gauze sponges.

C   The muscle incision has been completed. Note how the mucosa bulges. The incision extends onto the cardia of the stomach. The cranial extent of the esophageal incision varies with the surgeon, but it should extend onto the dilated portion of the esophagus. The incision site should be carefully examined to make sure all muscle fibers have been incised. The esophagus may be occluded above and below the mucosal incision and checked for mucosal leak by injecting saline.

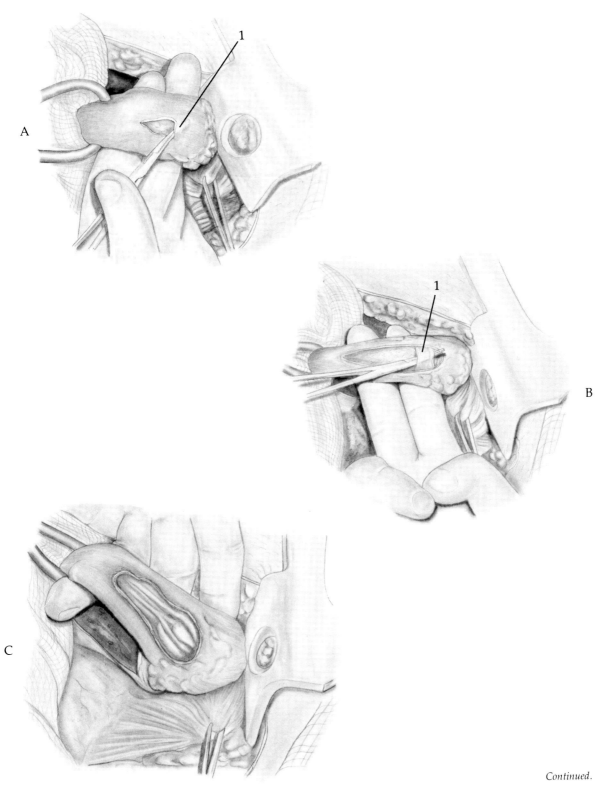

Continued.

PLATE 14

45

Plate 14. **Modified Heller procedure—cont'd**

D The esophagus is returned to the chest, and the cardia of the stomach is replaced into the abdomen. The sutures in the phrenoesophageal ligament *(1)* and diaphragm *(2)* are identified.

E The edge of the diaphragm *(1)* is grasped between the tagging sutures *(2)*. A nonabsorbable simple interrupted suture *(3)* is started between the tagging sutures *(2)* on the diaphragm, carried to the point of the incision of the esophageal muscularis *(4)*, and tied.

F The esophageal muscularis and phrenoesophageal ligament are sutured to the free edge of the diaphragm with simple interrupted sutures of nonabsorbable material.

If the esophageal hiatus is not closed properly, the stomach will be free to slide into the thorax, resulting in a diaphragmatic hernia. If the esophageal hiatus is closed too tightly, a stenosis of the esophagus could occur. The esophageal hiatal closure just described completely repairs the esophageal hiatus and at the same time widens the esophagus as it passes through the hiatus rather than produce a stenosis.

After repair of the esophageal hiatus, the chest is thoroughly lavaged with warm saline–povidone-iodine (Betadine) solution (Chapter 5), and the chest is closed with a chest tube in place (Chapter 3).

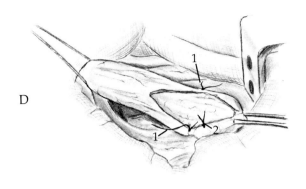

D

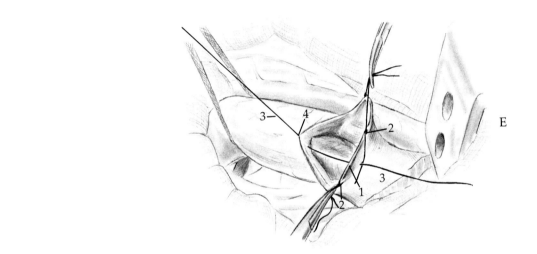

E

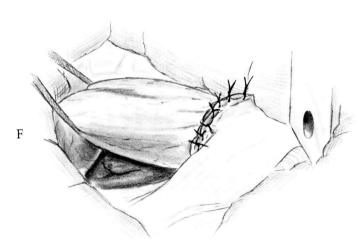

F

PLATE 14, cont'd

47

REFERENCES

Gourley, I. M. G., and Leighton, R. L.: Esopha-gotomy and pyloromyotomy in the dog, Pract. Vet. **43**:19, 1971.

Hoffer, R. E., Valdes-Da Pena, A., and Baue, A. E.: A comparative study of naturally occur-ring achalasia, Arch. Surg. **95**:83, 1967.

Hoffer, R. E.: Diseases of the esophagus. In Kirk, R. W., editor: Current veterinary therapy, vol. VI, Philadelphia, 1977, W. B. Saunders Co.

7
Lobectomy

The technique of lobectomy is used to remove a severely damaged non-functioning lung lobe. Neoplasia, chronic granuloma, infection with abscess, lung torsion, or lung trauma may all result in the need for lobectomy.

The technique to be described involves the removal of a lung lobe as a unit. The lung of the dog is divided into seven separate lobes, each supplied by its own vessels and bronchus. The seven lobes are the right and left cranial lobes, the right and left middle lobes, the right and left caudal lobes, and the right accessory lobe. If only a portion of the lobe is damaged, as may occur with trauma, partial lobectomy is possible.

Plate 15. Lobectomy

A The left chest has been entered at the sixth intercostal space. The left caudal lobe *(1)* is being retracted cranially, putting tension on the pulmonary ligament *(2)*. The aorta *(3)*, middle lobe *(4)*, and phrenic nerve *(5)* passing over the heart are seen. To expose the pulmonary vessels, the pulmonary ligament is carefully incised from its free edge *(6)* to its reflection onto the pulmonary vein *(7)*.

B The caudal lobe *(1)* has been reflected caudally and the mediastinum *(2)* cleaned from the pulmonary artery *(3)*. The left caudal pulmonary arterial branch *(4)* has been triple ligated. I prefer to ligate the artery first because this will prevent pooling of blood in the lobe to be removed. The vessel will be divided, leaving two ligatures on the proximal part of the artery. Some surgeons prefer to use a fixation ligature on these vessels. The left caudal pulmonary artery passes dorsal to the bronchus *(5)* and is the largest branch of the left pulmonary artery. The relationship of the other branches of the pulmonary arteries is well described in *Anatomy of the Dog.**

C The caudal lobe has been reflected dorsal/lateral to expose the pulmonary vein *(1)*. The number of pulmonary veins is variable as described in *Anatomy of the Dog*. The stump of the pulmonary artery *(2)* with its two ligatures is seen. A right-angle forceps has been passed between the pulmonary vein and the bronchus *(3)*. Note the bifurcation of the pulmonary vein *(4)*. The right-angle forceps is used to pass three ligatures around the vein.

D The pulmonary vein has been ligated and divided, leaving two ligatures close to the atrium.

---

*Miller, M. E., Christensen, G. C., and Evans, H. E.: Anatomy of the dog, Philadelphia, 1968, W. B. Saunders Co.

50

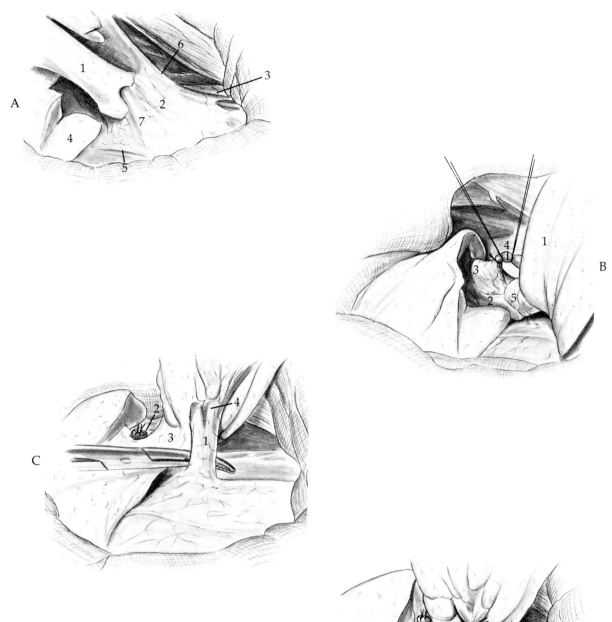

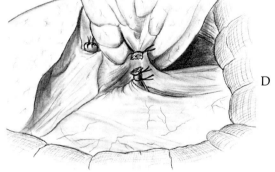

PLATE 15

Continued.

Plate 15.   Lobectomy—cont'd

E   The left caudal bronchus has been cleaned of its mediastinum and a bronchus clamp applied across it. The clamp should be placed close to the origin of this bronchus. The bronchus is being severed with scissors.

F   The left caudal lobe has been removed. The bronchus is being closed with a 4-0 nonabsorbable suture material in a simple interrupted suture pattern. These sutures are placed close together to appose the severed bronchus.

G   The bronchus has been closed *(1)*. The stumps of the pulmonary artery *(2)* and vein *(3)* are seen. Note the free border of the dissected mediastinum *(4)*. The surgical site is flushed with sterile saline solution. Saline is allowed to pool over the stump of the bronchus, and the stump is then observed for leaks. If any occur, they are closed with additional sutures. After the bronchus is sealed, the mediastinum is sutured loosely over the stump with absorbable sutures. The bronchus may also be closed with a crisscrossing simple interrupted suture pattern (Plate 10).

The thorax is thoroughly lavaged, the chest tube placed, and the thoracotomy closed (Chapter 3). The chest tube generally has to be left in position after lobectomy until all the space left by the excised lung lobe is filled by expansion of the remaining lobes. The tube can usually be removed 48 hours following lobectomy. If a unilateral pneumonectomy is done, the tube may have to remain for up to 72 hours.

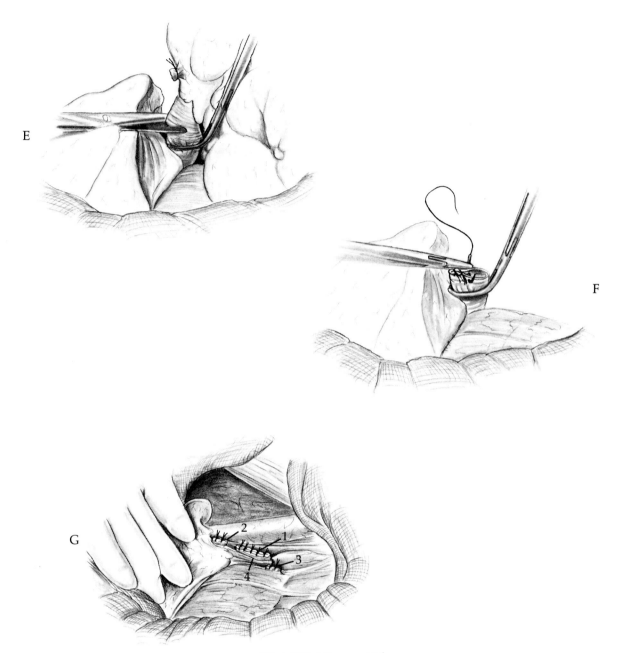

PLATE 15, cont'd

PART THREE
ABDOMEN

8
Abdominal exposures and closures

ABDOMINAL EXPOSURES

Incisions of the abdominal ventral midline may be divided into three areas: (1) the cranial ventral midline, which extends from the xiphoid to the umbilicus, (2) the middle ventral midline, which extends cranially and caudally from the umbilicus, and (3) the caudal ventral midline, which extends from the umbilicus to the pubis.

The incision to be described will be made through the linea alba. If the incision is made through the linea alba, bleeding is minimal. It should be noted that in the caudal abdomen the linea becomes very narrow and in some dogs is almost nonexistent.

Plate 16.   Abdominal exposure

A   An incision has been made from the xiphoid to the level of the umbilicus. The initial incision penetrates the skin *(1)* and subcutaneous tissue *(2)*, exposing the linea alba *(3)*. Bleeding is controlled by ligating vessels with 3-0 gut or electrocautery. The cranial superficial epigastric arteries at the xiphoid should be avoided. The subcutaneous tissue is being tensed by thumb forceps, and the scalpel is being used to reflect the subcutaneous tissue from the linea alba. The blade is held at a 45-degree angle, with the back on the abdominal wall. The blade is advanced, and the tissue is incised. It is important that traction be kept on the subcutaneous tissue while the incision is being made. Scissors may also be used to reflect the subcutaneous tissue.

B   The subcutaneous tissue *(1)* has been reflected, exposing the linea alba *(2)*. Note that the subcutaneous tissue is reflected only 1 to 2 mm on each side of the linea alba. Reflection of the subcutaneous tissue is especially important in the obese animal. Reflection permits easier closure of the muscle fascia by keeping fat out of the incision and allowing better visualization of the linea alba.

C   The middle ventral midline abdominal incision is shown. Note the umbilicus *(1)*.

D   The skin incision for a caudal ventral midline incision in the male dog is demonstrated, showing the skin incision lateral to the sheath *(1)*. The preputial muscle is severed by this incision. Note the vascular branches *(2)* from the external pudendal vessels. These vessels should be clamped, ligated, and divided. If the skin incision is extended to the pubis, it will be necessary to retract or to ligate and divide the external pudendal vessels.

In the male a thick fascial plane is encountered cranial to the sheath. This is sometimes distinct enough to be mistaken for the abdominal wall.

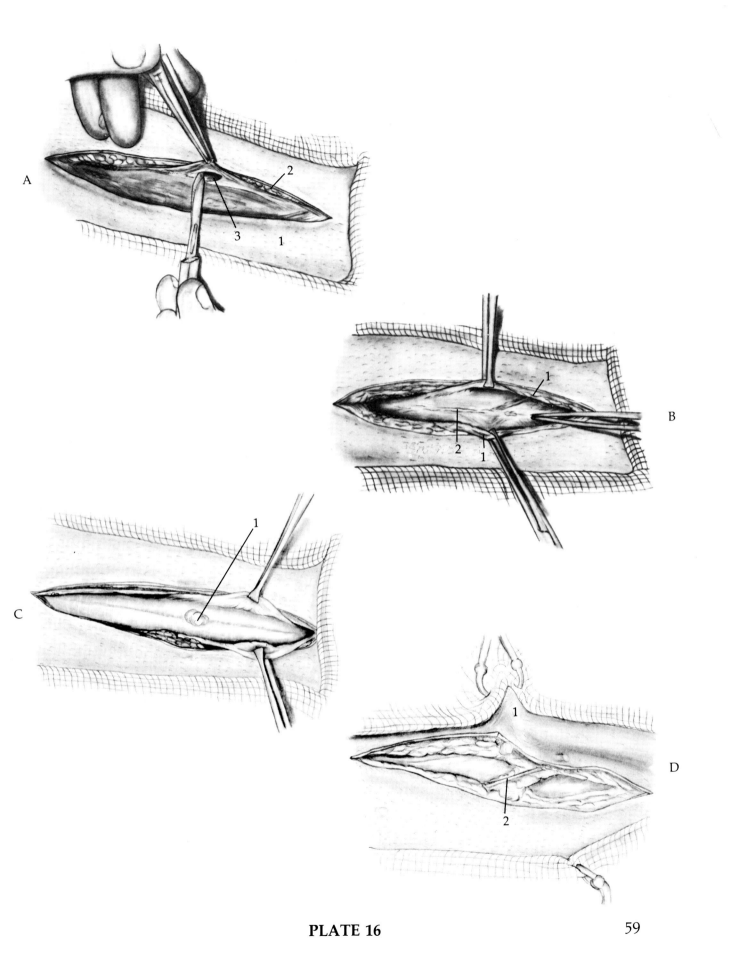

PLATE 16

Plate 17. Abdominal exposure

A The subcutaneous tissue *(1)* has been dissected from the abdominal wall and reflected medially, exposing the linea alba *(2)*. When this incision is being closed, the subcutaneous tissue has to be accurately apposed to eliminate dead space and to return the sheath to it normal position. In the male, if both sides of the penis are incised, paraphimosis may occur, since the function of both preputial muscles will be impaired. In the bitch the caudal incision is made on the ventral midline in the same manner that the cranial or middle incision is placed.

B To enter the abdomen the surgeon grasps the linea alba with toothed thumb forceps *(1)* and elevates it. The scalpel *(2)* is inserted into the tented portion of the linea with the blade directed straight forward. In this way the viscera will not be inadvertently damaged. If an animal has had previous abdominal surgery, the abdomen should not be initially entered along the old scar line because there may be adhesions of the viscera to the peritoneal scar.

C A thumb forceps *(1)* (or a grooved director) is inserted into the stab incision, and the linea is elevated. Then the linea is incised with the scalpel blade or scissors to complete the opening. If adhesions are a possibility, the incision should be done carefully. As soon as the incision is large enough, a finger is inserted and the intended incision site is palpated for adherent viscera.

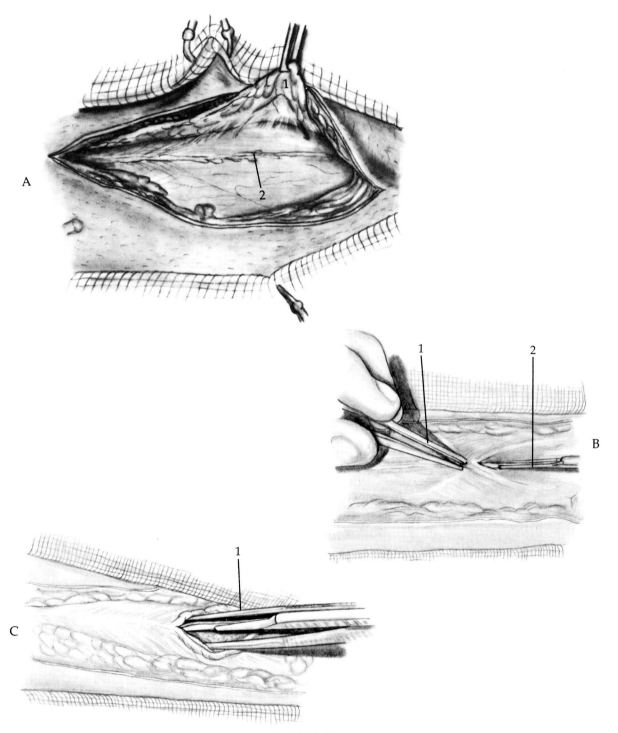

PLATE 17

Plate 18. Abdominal exposure

A   The entire abdomen has been opened without displacing the viscera. The falciform ligament *(1)* is seen covering the cranial aspect of the abdomen. A small portion of the spleen *(2)*, a loop of bowel *(3)*, and the tip of a partially distended bladder *(4)* are also seen.

B   The falciform ligament *(1)* has been removed from one side of the peritoneum and is being reflected laterally. The falciform ligament should be excised at this point, since if the falciform remains, it may interfere with anticipated surgical manipulations. The stomach *(2)*, spleen *(3)*, bowel *(4)*, and bladder *(5)* are better exposed after the removal of the falciform ligament.

C   The abdominal wall is being retracted to better expose the viscera. Note how the omentum *(1)* covers most of the viscera and attaches to the greater curvature of the stomach *(2)*.

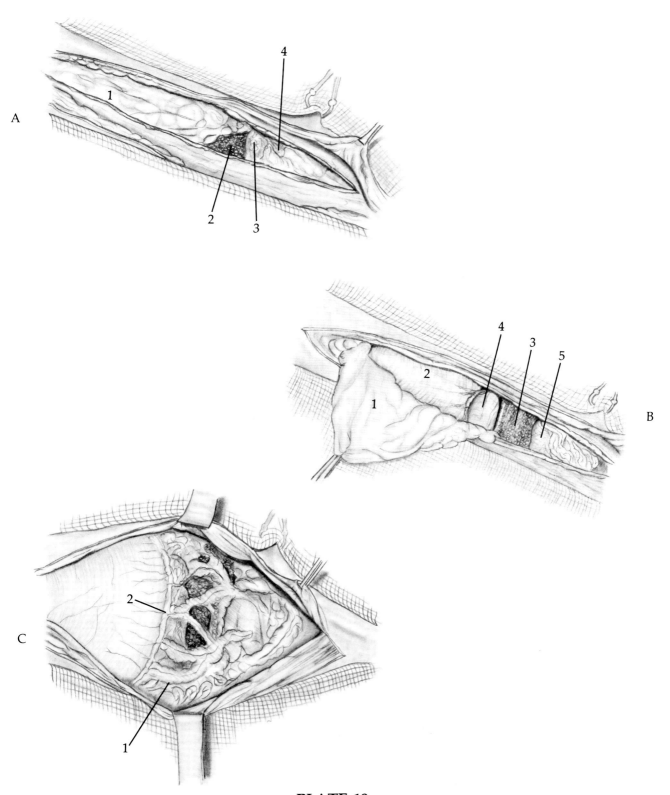

A

B

C

PLATE 18

Plate 19. Abdominal approach

A The omentum and spleen *(1)* have been reflected cranially, exposing the intestines *(2)* and urinary bladder *(3)*. In looking at this plate, keep in mind the areas of abdominal incision.

B The mesentery of the descending colon *(1)* is being used to pack off the abdominal viscera to expose the left kidney. The surgeon should be on the right side of the table to obtain the best exposure. The left kidney *(2)*, spermatic vessels *(3)*, ureter *(4)*, and vas deferens *(5)* can be clearly seen. The bladder *(6)* is being retracted caudally.

C The surgeon is on the left side of the table, and the descending duodenum mesentery *(1)* is being used to pack off the intestinal viscera to expose the right kidney *(2)*. Care should be taken not to traumatize the pancreas as it is reflected with the duodenum. The pancreas *(3)*, ureter *(4)*, spermatic vessels *(5)*, and vas deferens *(6)* can all be clearly visualized. Note the liver *(7)* lying on the cranial aspect of the right kidney.

This same method of exposure of the right and left kidneys is used to recover a dropped ovarian artery, as is discussed in Chapter 17. Details necessary for surgical manipulation of specific organs are discussed in the chapters relating to the surgery for those organs.

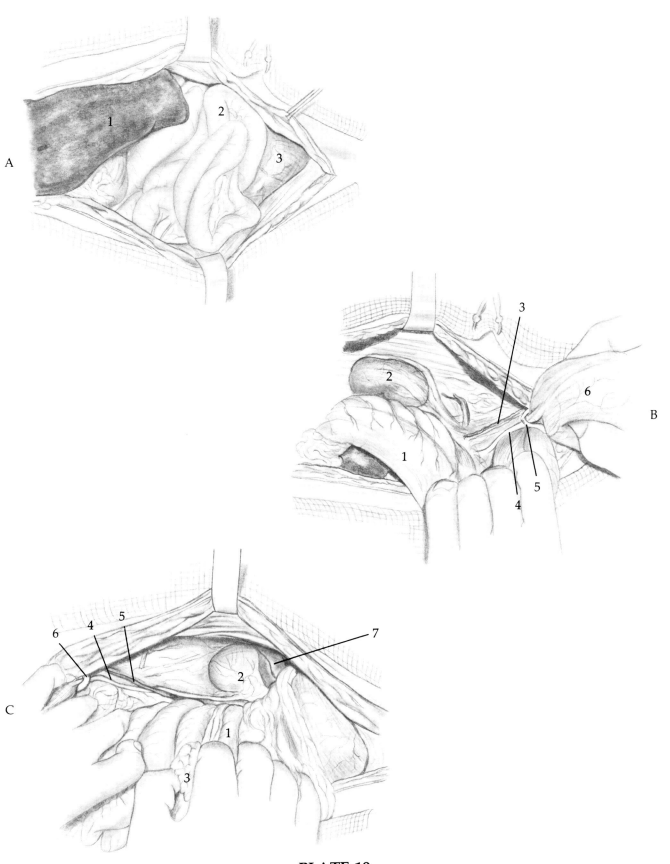

PLATE 19

65

ABDOMINAL CLOSURES

The surgeon may close the abdomen with three or four layers of sutures. A three-layer closure is satisfactory for most routine procedures. If the procedure has been lengthy or traumatic or the surgical area has been contaminated, then a four-layer closure is more satisfactory. If peritoneal lavage is anticipated, a four-layer closure should always be used. If the surgery was routine, absorbable suture material may be used for the buried layers. If contamination occurred, it is advisable to use nonabsorbable (wire) sutures when closing the muscle fascia.

Regardless of whether a four-layer or three-layer closure is used, the peritoneum must be apposed carefully. This allows an immediate fibrin seal of the abdomen. The muscle fascia or linea alba or both provide the strength of the abdominal closure. The subcutaneous closure eliminates dead space and is especially important in obese animals. The skin should be closed with nonabsorbable suture material in the pattern chosen by the surgeon. The skin closure should be cosmetically acceptable because this is the only part of the operation that the client sees.

Plate 20.   Abdominal closure

A   The four layers to be closed are the peritoneum (1), muscle fascia (2), subcutaneous tissue (3), and skin (4). The closure is being started at the xiphoid cartilage. The thumb forceps are grasping and reflecting the linea alba (5), a band of collagenous tissue that is the main insertion of the abdominal muscles. The peritoneum is also joined to the linea. If the opening incision has not been placed exactly through the linea alba, the peritoneum retracts from the midline. The surgeon must be sure to identify the retracted peritoneum and include it in the first layer of closure. In the caudal abdomen the linea becomes much narrower and the peritoneum thinner; therefore care must be taken to identify and pick up the caudal peritoneum.

B   The first suture (1) has been placed through the peritoneum. This suture is placed 2 mm lateral to the linea alba (2). The peritoneum (3) only is picked up.

C   The second bite of suture (1) is placed through the peritoneum (2) on the opposite side. Note the linea alba (3). This suture is tied, and the remainder of the peritoneum is closed with a simple continuous peritoneal suture to the end of the incision, where it is tied. It is important that the extreme ends of the peritoneal incision be sutured. This may be accomplished by starting and ending the peritoneal suture in intact peritoneum.

D   The muscle fascia or linea alba (1) is closed with a simple interrupted suture pattern with the sutures 3 to 4 mm apart. Note how the peritoneal closure (2) has everted the linea alba. This method produces two peritoneal appositions if the opening incision was made directly through the linea alba.

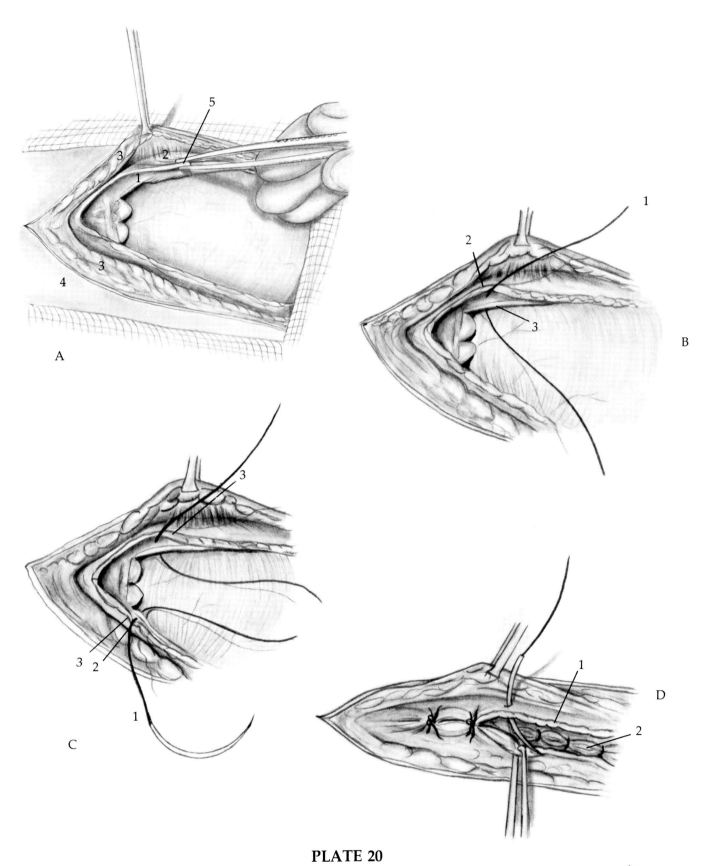

PLATE 20

Plate 21.   Abdominal closure

A   The first layer of a three-layer closure is begun by inserting the needle through the muscle fascia and peritoneum lateral to the linea alba *(1)*.

B   The suture is passed through the other side of the incision. Note that the suture emerges lateral to the linea alba *(1)*. When these sutures are being placed, the linea alba should be everted so that the peritoneum is visible. By doing this, the surgeon will always include the peritoneum in the suture pattern. The linea alba sutures are tied *(2)*, apposing the peritoneum and muscle fascia with a single layer of simple interrupted sutures. The ends of the incision should be tightly closed and should be checked by the surgeon before closing the subcutaneous tissue. The linea alba sutures or muscle fascia sutures should not include muscle per se. Muscle tissue has very little holding power and consequently will not increase the strength of the closure. Also, muscle may undergo necrosis when sutured, resulting in pain at the incision site that could cause self-mutilation by the patient. The subcutaneous tissue is apposed with simple interrupted sutures *(3)*. Some surgeons prefer to close the subcutaneous layer with a simple continuous suture. As mentioned in caudal abdominal exposure, the tissue under the sheath and the preputial muscles must be apposed by the subcutaneous tissue sutures. The skin has been closed with a simple interrupted suture *(4)*. This may be placed using a surgeon's knot. The first throw of the knot apposes the skin edges. The second throw is not tightened, leaving a 1 mm loop on top of the first throw. The third throw is tightened on top of the second throw. This allows the first throw to expand when the skin swells and prevents the knots from becoming too tight. Modifications of skin closures, such as a stent pack or Penrose drain, are described in other chapters.

C   When the abdomen has been contaminated, the technique of intermittent peritoneal lavage may be helpful. The decision as to whether to use it should be made before closing because placement of the lavage tube is easier when the abdomen is open. Silastic medical-grade 1/4-inch O.D. tubing is used for this technique. A small incision *(1)* is made 5 cm lateral and 6 cm cranial or caudal to the area of the abdomen where the tube is to be placed. Generally the tube is placed cranial for a caudal abdominal incision and caudal for a cranial abdominal incision. An attempt should be made to place the tip of the tube next to the damaged organ if it is a fixed organ such as the pancreas. If the abdomen is generally contaminated, as from bowel spillage, this is not necessary. A Carmalt forceps is passed subcutaneously *(2)* and forced through the abdominal wall. The tube *(4)* is grasped by the forceps, and the forceps and tube are withdrawn.

D   The tube *(1)* has been withdrawn through the abdominal wall, leaving a length of tube in the abdomen for drainage. Note the precut holes *(2)* in the tube.

After the tube has been put in place, the abdomen should be completely lavaged with warm sterile saline solution and aspirated dry. If there was abdominal contamination, the abdomen is then lavaged with a solution of 15 ml of povidone-iodine (Betadine Whirlpool Concentrate) in 1000 ml of saline and aspirated dry. The abdomen is then closed. The tube is fixed to the skin as described for fixing a chest tube (Chapter 3).

Intermittent lavage, if necessary, is begun 24 hours after the abdomen is closed, which allows time for the peritoneum to seal. Lavage is repeated two to three times a day. The reader is referred to the references for detailed information on peritoneal lavage.

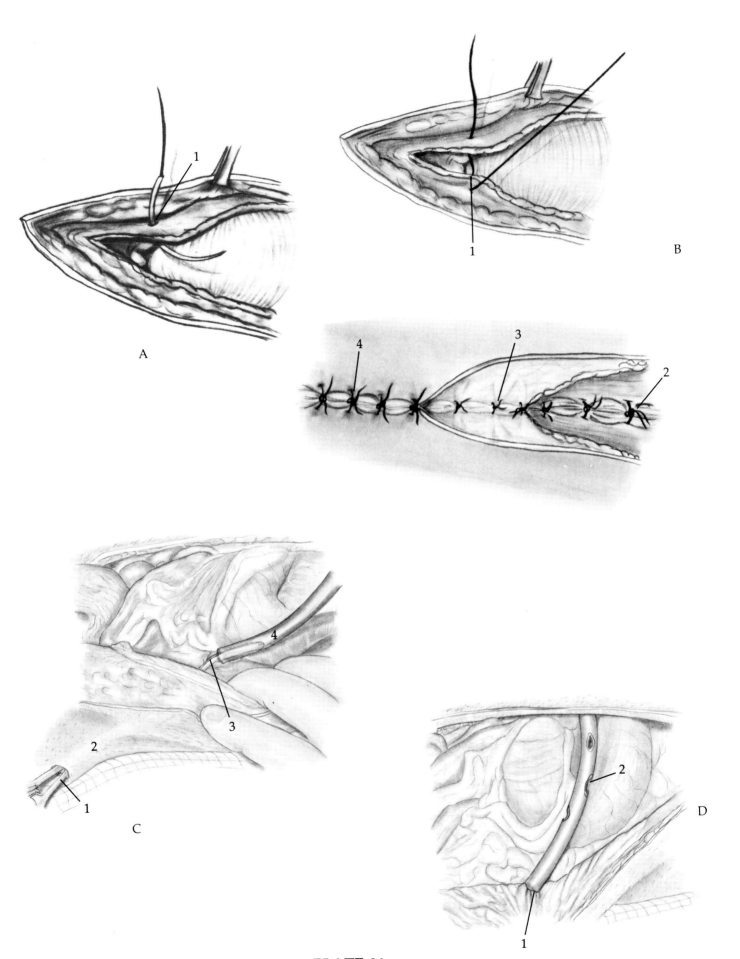

A

B

C

D

PLATE 21

REFERENCES

Hoffer, R. E.: Peritonitis, Vet. Clin. North Am. **2**:189, 1972.

Hoffer, R. E.: The peritoneum. In Bojrab, M. J.: Current techniques in small animal surgery, Philadelphia, 1975, Lea & Febiger.

9
Diaphragmatic hernia repair

A diaphragmatic hernia occurs as the result of a defect in the diaphragm or its attachments that allows abdominal viscera to invade the thoracic cavity. The defect is most commonly the result of trauma, although congenital diaphragmatic defects are occasionally seen.

Most traumatic hernias involve a tear not only of the muscular crura of the diaphragm but also of portions of the ventral and lateral attachments of the crura to the ribs and sternum. The diaphragmatic defect may involve the vena caval hiatus, esophageal hiatus, or aortic hiatus. If these structures are involved, care must be exercised when closing the defect not to damage or partially occlude them.

Hydrothorax is often associated with diaphragmatic hernia. Generally these patients are in severe respiratory distress when presented and require extremely careful induction of anesthesia with assisted ventilation.

The object of surgery is to replace the abdominal viscera and restore the integrity of the diaphragm.

There are three common approaches used for diaphragmatic hernia repair. A right or left caudal thoracotomy may be used, providing the hernia is on the right or the left side exclusively. I prefer to use a cranial ventral midline abdominal approach (Chapter 8). This approach exposes the entire diaphragm, and any type of diaphragmatic defect can be repaired. If the hernia is of long standing and thoracic adhesions are present, the sternum can be partially split to give more thoracic exposure; this is rarely necessary.

Plate 22.   Diaphragmatic hernia

A   The abdomen has been opened, exposing the hernia in the right crura. Allis tissue forceps (1) have been placed on the diaphragmatic tear. Part of the liver (2) is in the diaphragmatic defect. The stomach (3) is caudal to the liver. If hydrothorax is present, a suction apparatus should be available. If suction is not available, towels or large sponges may be utilized to remove the excess fluid.

B   The liver and abdominal viscera have been removed from the thorax. The edges of the diaphragmatic tear (1) can be clearly seen. The liver (2) is reflected caudally, exposing the vena caval hiatus (3). Note that the defect has completely exposed the vena cava (4). The lung (5) can be seen alongside the vena cava. The liver may be easily ruptured if excessive traction is placed on it while it is being removed from the thorax. Therefore it may be necessary to enlarge the diaphragmatic defect to avoid damaging the liver while it is being manipulated.

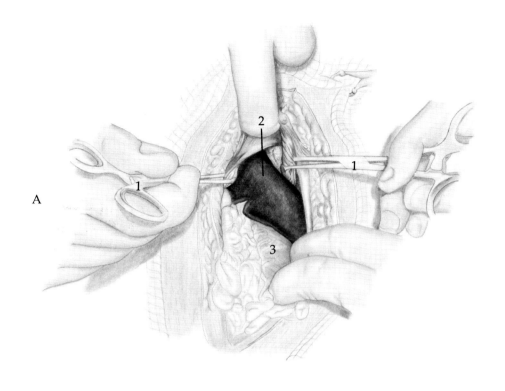

A

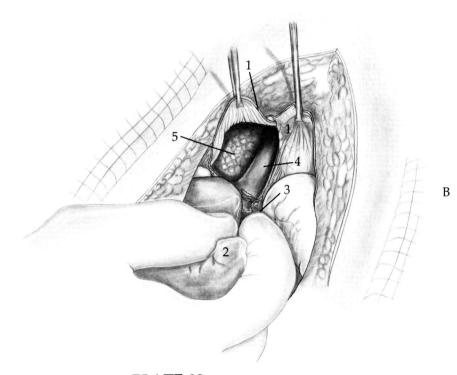

B

PLATE 22

73

Plate 23. Diaphragmatic hernia

A The area around the vena cava is closed first. Two or three preplaced simple interrupted sutures *(1)* of 0 medium chromic gut have been placed through the edges of the diaphragmatic tear. These sutures should be carefully placed to avoid perforating the vena cava. Traction is applied to the sutures, closing the vena caval hiatus. The vena cava is examined to be certain that it is not occluded. If the cava is compromised, the sutures are removed and placed so the hiatus is not closed as tightly. Closing the vena caval hiatus is the most important part of the procedure.

B The first suture *(1)* has been tied. One end is left long for traction. The second suture *(2)* has been tied. This suture serves as the start for the simple continuous pattern used to close the remainder of the diaphragmatic defect. A chest tube (Chapter 3) should be placed before the remaining diaphragmatic defect is closed. Note that the lungs *(3)* have been fully expanded. The mediastinum should also be broken down to permit free drainage of the chest.

C The diaphragmatic tear has been closed with a simple continuous suture of 0 chromic gut *(1)*. The suture incorporates large bites of the muscular crura. This is necessary to obtain a good strong closure. Note the suture *(2)* that was preplaced at the vena caval hiatus. The suture is finished below the xiphoid cartilage, and this is included in the suture pattern to completely seal the defect. The chest tube is seen *(3)*.

If the diaphragm had been torn from the rib attachments, the same suture pattern would be used. The suture may be passed around the ribs for added strength.

If the edges of the diaphragmatic defect appear to be healed, the edges should be freshened before suturing them.

The abdomen is closed (Chapter 8). The chest tube is aspirated as described in Chapter 3. Systemic antibiotics are administered for the first 5 days. The chest tube can generally be removed after 24 hours. The dog is started on food and water very slowly to prevent any vomiting.

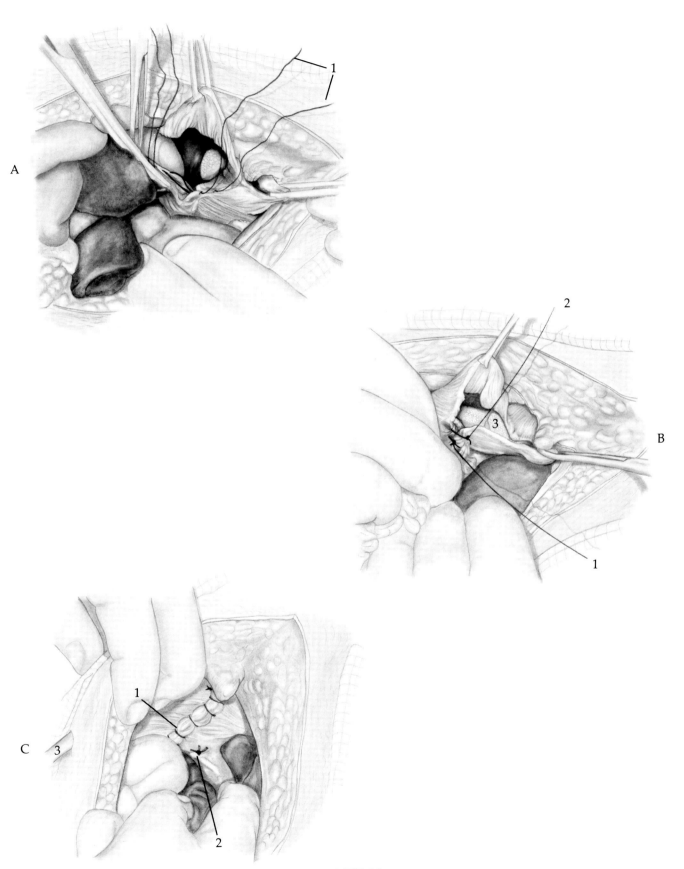

PLATE 23

REFERENCE

Wilson, G. P., Newton, C. D., and Burt, J. K.: A review of 116 diaphragmatic hernias in dogs and cats, J. Am. Vet. Med. Assoc. **159**:1142, 1971.

10
Gastrotomy

Gastrotomy is performed primarily to remove a foreign body from the stomach. It also may used to explore the stomach for evidence of neoplasia, ulceration, or pyloric stenosis.

The abdomen is entered via a cranial ventral midline incision (Chapter 8). The stomach can usually be seen on entry to the abdomen. The stomach is grasped either with Allis tissue forceps or digitally and pulled through the incision. The stomach is then examined visually and by palpation to locate the foreign body or the lesion. The pylorus should also be examined.

If the patient has a history of eating objects or if the clinical signs indicate that probability, the intestinal tract should be palpated to see if there are any additional foreign bodies. If neoplasia is suspected, the lymph nodes in the area should be examined. Even if the lymph nodes appear normal, they should be biopsied.

Plate 24.   Gastrotomy

A   After the exploration the ventral body of the stomach is exteriorized with two Allis tissue forceps *(1)*. The forceps are placed midway between the lesser and greater curvatures of the body of the stomach. This can be determined by observing where the branches from the gastric and gastroepiploic vessels anastomose *(2)*. This is the least vascular portion of the stomach. The stomach is packed off with a saline-soaked towel. If possible, the foreign body is exteriorized with the stomach. Note the small impressions on the stomach *(3)*. These are caused by pressure from the gastric foreign body. An incision is made into the lumen of the stomach. This may be done by putting tension on the Allis tissue forceps and quickly, with a stabbing action of the scalpel, penetrating all the layers of the stomach. The incision is enlarged with scissors to the length necessary to perform the manipulations.

B   The mucosa *(1)* will separate from the seromuscular layer *(2)*. Note the foreign body *(3)* beginning to emerge through the incision. The incision should be large enough to permit easy removal of any foreign object without tearing the incision. If exploration of the gastric lumen is necessary, the incision should also permit this easily. The gastric lumen may be digitally explored if the foreign object is small or if more than one object is present. Enlarging the gastric incision will expose the lumen and allow a biopsy of a mucosal mass to be obtained.

If the stomach is full at the time of surgery, suctioning at the time of the initial stab incision will evacuate the contents without excessive contamination of the area.

78

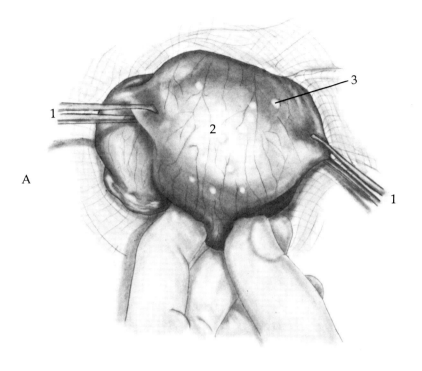

A

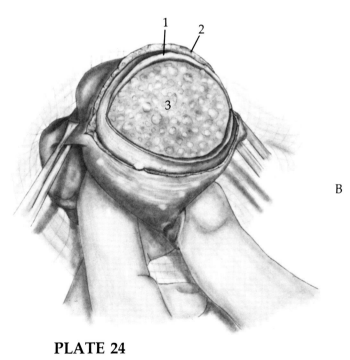

B

PLATE 24

Plate 25. Gastrotomy

A   The gastric incision is closed with a two-layer suture pattern and 3-0 chromic gut with a swaged noncutting needle. A Connell-Halsted suture pattern is described, but the stomach may be closed with any combination of inverting sutures. The Connell suture pattern is started in the seromuscular layer just past the incision site (1). A simple interrupted suture is placed and tied, leaving the end long (2). The needle is inserted through the stomach wall from outside to inside on the upper aspect of the incision (3). The needle is next inserted from inside to outside on the upper aspect and parallel to the incision (4). This may be accomplished with one motion.

B   The suture is passed directly across to the lower aspect of the incision (1) and inserted in this portion in the same manner. Note the loop of suture in the lumen (2).

C   Observe the way the suture is advanced; it penetrates all stomach layers. This illustration demonstrates a point. Normally the suture line is tightened each time the needle is removed.

D   To finish the suture pattern the last bite of the needle (1) is placed so it emerges past the incision on one side. The entire suture line is tightened until the edges of the incision are completely inverted.

E   The needle is passed through the seromuscular layer in a simple interrupted pattern (1). This forms a loop (2). Note the complete inversion of the edges of the incision.

F   The free end of the suture is tied to the loop (1), thus completing the Connell suture pattern.

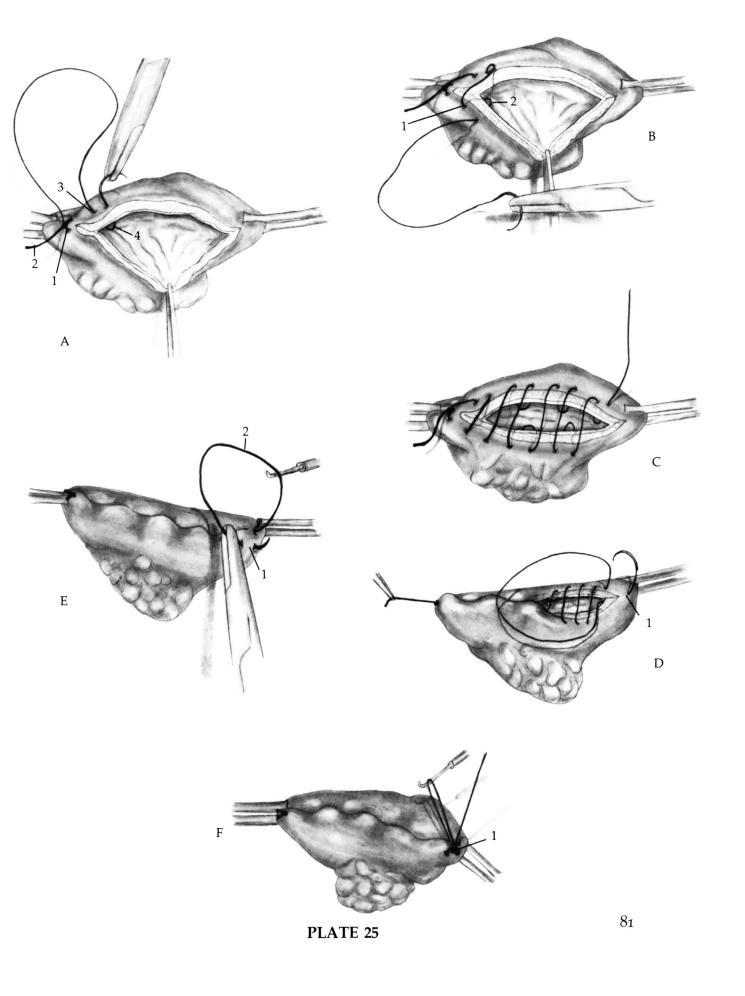

PLATE 25

Plate 26. Gastrotomy

A A Halsted suture pattern is placed in the second layer. This may also be of 3-0 chromic gut with a swaged needle. The needle is inserted through the seromuscular layer to the submucosa on the far side of the incision *(1)*. The submucosa can be felt by the tip of the needle. It feels firm and is difficult to penetrate. The needle is brought out on the same side of the incision, as if placing a simple interrupted suture. This suture should be placed close to the first layer of sutures and should not penetrate the mucosa. The needle is placed on the near side of the incision with the same technique *(2)*. The needle is now reversed, and the submucosa is penetrated on the near side of the incision *(3)*. The same technique is used on the far side of the incision *(4)*.

B The suture is tied, producing serosa-to-serosa contact. Note that the first Halsted suture *(1)* has inverted the knot that finished the Connell suture. The last suture inverts the knot that started the Connell suture *(2)*. The entire Connell suture line has been inverted. The amount of tissue inverted is determined by the distance the suture is placed from the incision, and the smaller the amount of tissue included in the suture on each side of the incision, the smaller the amount of tissue inverted.

When the closure is completed, the surgical site is rinsed with sterile saline solution, and the towel packing is removed. The abdomen may be lavaged if contamination occurred. Also, a lavage tube may be utilized (Chapter 8). The instruments used for the gastrotomy are discarded. The operating stand and patient are redraped, and the surgeon changes gloves and gown.

The abdomen is closed (Chapter 8). Antibiotics may be administered if contamination is suspected. The dog may be started on a liquid diet 24 hours postoperatively, provided there is no ileus. The patient may receive semisolid food by the third postoperative day and solid food by the seventh postoperative day.

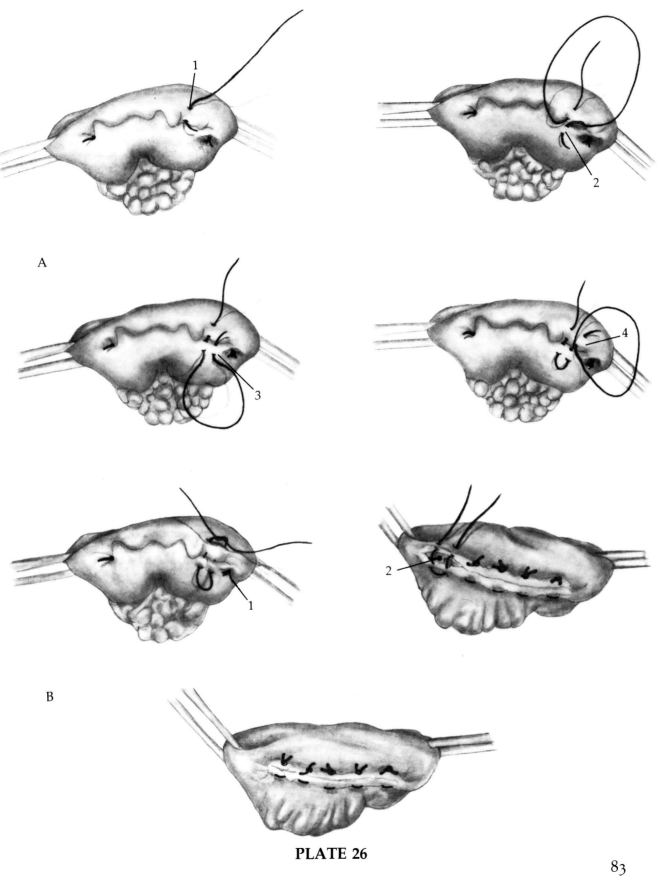

A

B

PLATE 26

11
Pyloric surgery—pyloromyotomy and pyloroplasty

Pyloric surgery is classically performed to relieve obstruction caused by hypertrophic pyloric stenosis. However, pyloric surgery may also be performed to decrease the emptying time of the stomach, to eliminate pyloric spasm, and to eliminate stricture produced by a foreign body damaging the pyloric sphincter.

There are two primary types of surgical manipulation of the pyloric sphincter. The first is pyloromyotomy, in which the muscles of the pyloric sphincter are incised without penetrating the mucosa. This is primarily used for hypertrophic pyloric stenosis or pyloric spasm. The second type of surgery is pyloroplasty, in which the configuration of the pyloric sphincter is changed.

If during a pyloromyotomy the mucosa is inadvertently damaged, the operation can easily be converted to a pyloroplasty to obtain the same end result. The advantage of the pyloromyotomy is that the lumen of the pylorus is not invaded. However, if the problem requiring pyloric surgery cannot definitely be proved to be caused only by abnormal musculature or function, a pyloroplasty is indicated. A pyloroplasty will permit the surgeon to visualize the mucosa of the pylorus. Thus, if there is redundant hypertrophied mucosal tissue, it can be removed.

85

Plate 27. Pyloromyotomy

A The pylorus is approached by a cranial ventral midline incision (Chapter 8). The stomach *(1)* and duodenum *(2)* are retracted caudoventrally. This draws the liver *(3)* caudally and exposes the pylorus *(4)*. The traction exposes the attachments of the lesser omentum from the duodenum to the liver (the hepatoduodenal ligament, *5)* and from the stomach to the liver (the hepatogastric ligament, *6)*. Although the common bile duct runs in the hepatoduodenal ligament, this is not always visible unless bile is flowing through it. The approach used so far is for either the pyloromyotomy or pyloroplasty. Care should be taken not to damage the pancreas while applying traction *(7)*.

B The initial longitudinal incision for pyloromyotomy is placed midway between the antimesenteric side and the mesenteric side of the pyloric sphincter. The incision should extend slightly cranial and caudal to the sphincter onto the stomach and duodenum. This can be determined by palpation.

C The initial incision has been made but is not completely through the musculature. Note that the circular muscles still cover the mucosa *(1)*.

D The mucosa has been exposed by hemostat dissection *(1)*. Scissors have been inserted under the circular fibers of the sphincter *(2)*. Care should be taken at this point, since it is easy to damage the mucosa while incising the muscle fibers covering it.

E All the muscle fibers have been incised, allowing the mucosa *(1)* to bulge out of the incision. It is important that all muscle fibers be incised so that there is no possibility of regrowth of the sphincter.

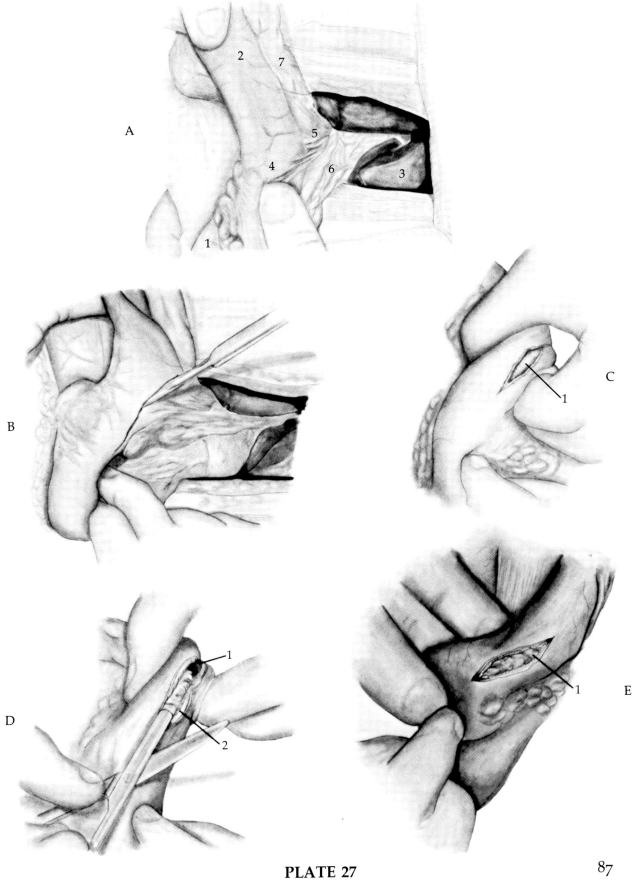

PLATE 27

87

Plate 28. Pyloroplasty

The pyloroplasty is performed by making a longitudinal incision through the pyloric sphincter and suturing it transversely. The basic suture pattern is the same as that described for closing an enterotomy (Chapter 12).

A The mucosa has been incised in preparation for pyloroplasty. If during a pyloromyotomy the mucosa is perforated, the mucosa should be incised and a pyloroplasty performed. Before a pyloromyotomy is converted to a pyloroplasty, intestinal forceps should be placed on the stomach and the duodenum. The operative area should then be packed off with sterile saline-soaked towels. If the surgeon elected initially to do a pyloroplasty, the beginning incision demonstrated in Plate 27, *B,* would be carried through the mucosa without undermining the muscularis.

B Note the thickness and redundancy of the mucosa as compared to **A.** This dog had pyloric stenosis secondary to mucosal hypertrophy.

C A nonabsorbable 5-0 suture has been placed through the mucosa and submucosa. Note that the suture is placed at the corners of the pyloric incision *(1).*

D The suture is tied, converting the longitudinal incision to a transverse closure. This suture *(1)* will be used to close the far side of the incision. Note that the tied end is left long *(2).*

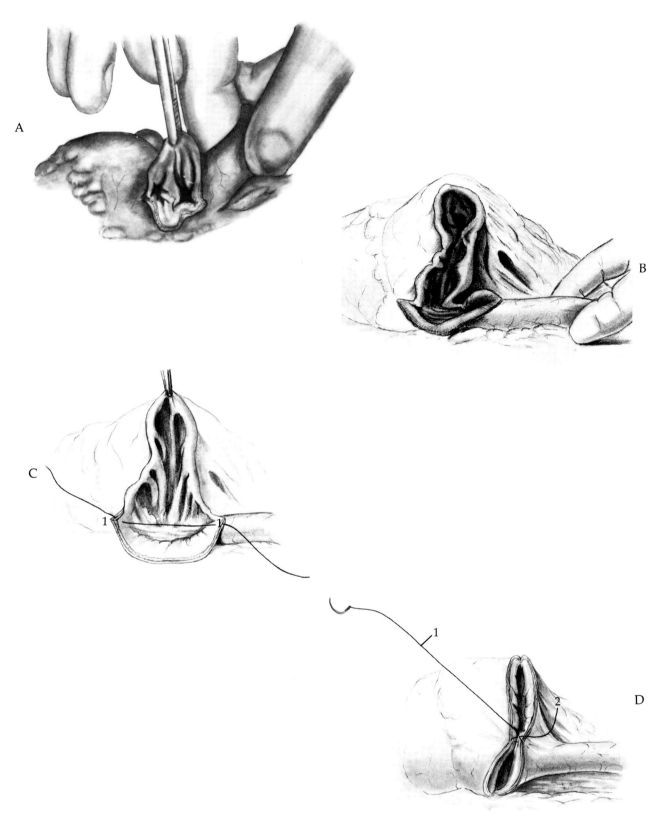

PLATE 28

Plate 29. Pyloroplasty

A The mucosa and submucosa are apposed on the far side *(1)* using a simple continuous suture pattern. The sutures are left loose in this plate to demonstrate the pattern. Normally, the sutures are drawn tight as placed. Note the long suture end *(2)* and that the near side continuous suture *(3)* is started at the near corner of the incision.

B The near side *(1)* is sutured to the middle of the incision with a simple continuous pattern. This suture is finished by tying it *(2)* to the long end *(3)* of the far side suture.

C The second layer is closed with a Halsted suture pattern of 3-0 absorbable suture *(1)*. Note that the Halsted suture is placed so that it will invert the knot from the continuous suture. The Halsted suture penetrates the seromuscular layer and picks up some of the submucosa. These sutures are placed close to the edge of the incision to prevent inversion of an excessive amount of tissue.

D The Halsted suture pattern has been completed. Note that all the knots from the first layer of sutures have been inverted. Note also that there is no mucosal protrusion through the second layer. The Halsted sutures at the corners of the incision have to be carefully placed to prevent mucosal protrusion. At the far corner it is best to preplace the last two or three Halsted sutures to allow good inversion of the mucosa.

If a pyloromyotomy has been done, the pylorus is returned to the abdomen and the abdomen closed. Food and water are withheld until gut motility returns. The dog may then be fed a bland diet for a few days.

If pyloroplasty has been done, the pylorus is rinsed and the towels removed. Contaminated instruments are discarded. The dog is redraped, and the surgeon's gloves and gown are changed before closing the abdomen. Appropriate antibiotics are administered if necessary. The abdomen is closed (Chapter 8). The postoperative feeding regimen is the same as for gastrotomy (Chapter 10). Peritoneal lavage may be utilized if contamination occurred (Chapter 8).

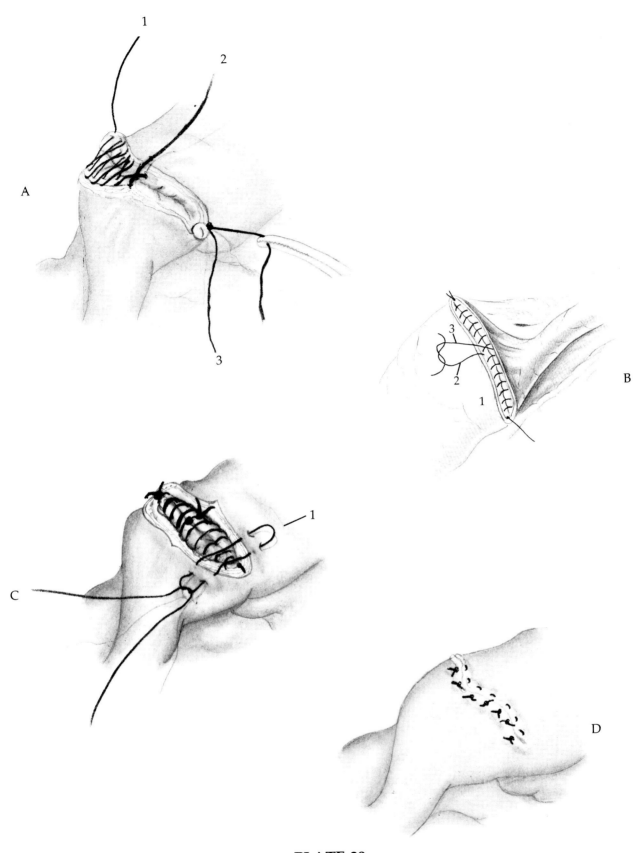

PLATE 29

REFERENCE

Harkins, H. N., Moyer, C. A., Rhoads, J. E., and
    Allen, J. G.: Surgery principles and practice, ed.
    2, Philadelphia, 1961, J. B. Lippincott Co.

12
Enterotomy

An enterotomy is performed to remove an obstructing object from the intestine. Before performing an enterotomy the surgeon must locate the obstruction. It must be remembered that occasionally more than one foreign body can be present in the bowel, and for this reason the entire gastrointestinal tract should be palpated and examined when an obstruction is to be removed. Generally the bowel will be distended with gas cranial to the obstruction and appear flaccid below it. After locating the obstruction, the surgeon must decide whether the obstructed bowel is viable. A viable bowel will be pink, appear moist, and not be excessively friable. A nonviable bowel will be dark blue to black, appear dry, and be very friable.

If there is any question as to the viability of the bowel, a resection and anastomosis should be performed rather than an enterotomy. The abdomen is opened with a midventral midline incision (Chapter 8).

Plate 30.   Enterotomy

A   After the obstruction has been found, it is exteriorized and packed off from the abdomen with saline-soaked towels *(1)*. Intestinal forceps are applied above and below the area to be incised *(2)*. The forceps may or may not be rubber shod. They should be tightened just enough to obstruct the flow of intestinal contents and should be left in position only while the lumen of the bowel is open.

B   The incision into the bowel is made on the antimesenteric side. The incision may be made over the object. However, if the intestine over the object appears abnormal, the incision should be made cranial to the mass to be removed. The cranial incision allows easier removal of the object, since this portion of the bowel is generally more distended than the caudal portion. After the initial incision has been made, the object may be grasped with forceps or a hemostat *(1)* and removed. Gentle digital pressure below the object will help remove it. The incision should be large enough to permit removal without tearing the incision site. If there is any indication that the incision is being stressed, the incision should be enlarged.

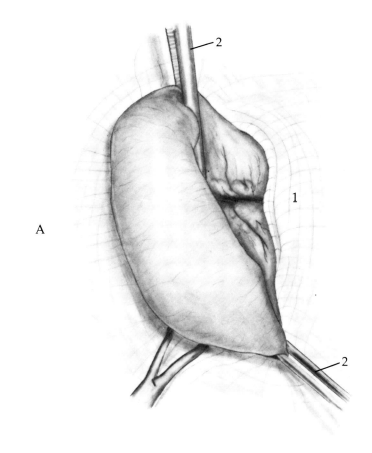

A

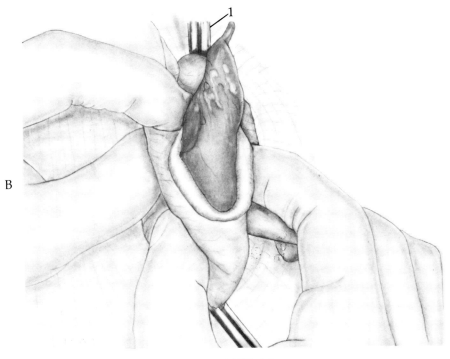

B

PLATE 30

Plate 31. Enterotomy

A The intestinal incision is closed by placing a simple continuous suture of 5-0 silk with a swaged needle through the edge of the mucosa and a portion of the submucosa. The sutures should be close to the edges of the mucosa and should evenly appose the mucosa. The needle is initially placed through the mucosa and submucosa at the end of the incision *(1)* so that it penetrates unincised mucosa. This suture is tied, and the simple continuous suture is continued from this point. Note that the suture penetrates only the mucosa and submucosa *(2)*.

B The simple continuous suture is finished by making the final suture and tie past the end of the mucosal incision. This is accomplished by passing the needle through the mucosa and submucosa 1 mm past the corner of the incision and typing this loop to itself *(1)*. While the simple continuous suture is being placed, it is important that tension be maintained on the suture line. This prevents the sutures from becoming loose, resulting in leakage in the suture line. After completion of the mucosal suture the suture line may be tested by injecting sterile saline solution into the lumen of the bowel and applying pressure. If there are any areas that leak, these may be repaired with a simple interrupted suture. The mucosal suture line should be tight before the second layer is closed. The second layer is closed with a Halsted suture *(2)* of 3-0 absorbable suture with a swaged needle. This suture penetrates the serosa, muscularis, and submucosa. The suture is placed close to the edge of the incision to prevent inversion of any more tissue than is necessary and yet to obtain a good closure. The Halsted suture is placed in the same manner as described for gastrotomy closure (Chapter 10). The needle is inserted into the submucosa and emerges on the same side *(3)*. The needle is brought to the opposite side of the incision, and the submucosa is picked up *(4)*. The needle is then reversed and penetrates the submucosa on the same side *(5)*. The needle is carried across the incision and again is inserted into the submucosa *(6)*.

C The sutures are tied, producing a serosa-to-serosa apposition without excess inversion of tissue *(1)*. Note that the Halsted sutures extend cranial and caudal to the mucosal suture line. Note also that there is no excessive narrowing of the sutured area of the bowel.

The bowel is rinsed with sterile saline solution and returned to the abdominal cavity. If the surgeon desires, omentum may be placed over the sutured area. At this point all instruments used during the enterotomy are discarded. The operating stand and patient are redraped, and the surgeon's gown and gloves are changed.

If contamination of the abdomen occurred during surgical manipulation or was present preoperatively, the abdomen should be thoroughly flushed with saline, a lavage tube should be placed (Chapter 8), and appropriate antibiotics should be administered.

Postoperatively the dog should be supported by parenteral fluids for 24 hours or until the paralytic ileus has regressed. This may be determined by seeing defecation or by auscultation of peristaltic sounds in the abdomen. Initially the dog is frequently given water in very small amounts so that vomiting does not occur. Liquids such as Esbilac may be given after the initial water. The dog should be on a semisolid diet by the third postoperative day. Full feeding may be resumed by the seventh postoperative day.

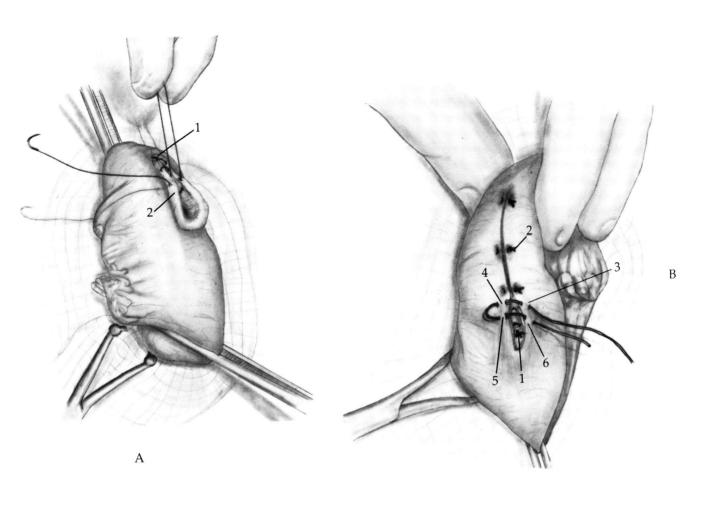

A

B

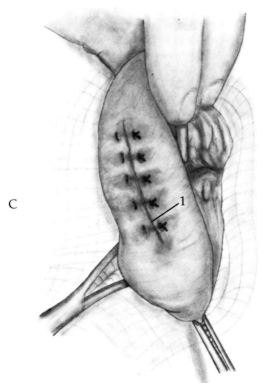

C

PLATE 31

13
Intestinal resection and anastomosis

Three techniques of intestinal anastomosis will be presented. A two-layer technique that utilizes end-to-end apposition of the mucosa and inversion of the serosa will be described first. The second technique will produce a two-layer end-to-end apposition of the mucosa with end-to-end inversion of the serosa with only a single layer of sutures. The third technique produces end-to-end apposition of all layers with a single row of sutures. Variations of techniques permitting end-to-end apposition of lumens of different diameters will also be described.

The basic technique of resection is the same for all methods of anastomosis.

Intestinal resection and anastomosis is performed to remove devitalized bowel and to reestablish functional bowel continuity. The resection should remove all devitalized bowel, leaving only viable bowel with a good blood supply for anastomosis. The anastomosis should produce a union that does not leak or constrict after surgery.

As mentioned previously (Chapter 12), surgery for an intestinal obstruction requires that the entire gastrointestinal tract be examined visually and palpated for evidence of multiple obstructions.

Manipulation of the bowel predisposes to the development of shock. Therefore the patient should be closely observed for impending shock and treated immediately. Preoperative therapy with corticosteroids, fluids, and antibiotics is of value in reducing the incidence of shock during bowel surgery.

If surgery of the colon is anticipated, enemas should be given prior to the operation, presupposing that the condition of the animal permits. To prevent postoperative infection, preoperative oral antibiotic therapy to sterilize the bowel is also of value.

Close attention to aseptic technique, adequate packing off of viscera, and careful handling of the bowel will all reduce the incidence of postoperative infection and peritonitis.

The techniques for resecting and anastomosing the jejunum will be described. The same basic principles of resection apply to the duodenum, ileum, and colon. The surgeon should remember that the blood supply to each area of the bowel is distributed differently. The reader is referred to *Anatomy of the Dog* for a review of the blood supply of the bowel.

Plate 32. Two-layer resection and anastomosis

A   A loop of jejunum has been exteriorized. Note the distribution of the jejunal arteries. The devitalized segment of the bowel is seen *(1)*. When a portion of the jejunum is to be removed, the intestinal blood supply should be occluded alongside a major jejunal artery *(2)* not associated with the diseased portion of the bowel. The jejunal arteries anastomose, forming an arcade *(3)* close to the mesenteric border of the bowel. From this arcade the vasa recti *(4)* go directly to the intestine, bifurcate, and encircle the gut. The diseased segment of bowel and the bowel to be anastomosed are packed off from the abdomen with saline-soaked towels.

B   A mosquito forceps *(1)* has been passed through the mesentery *(2)* between the terminal arcade and the intestinal wall. This is facilitated by staying right on the intestinal wall with the hemostat. The forceps is opened, stripping the mesentery away from the intestinal wall and creating an opening of 0.5 cm between the arcade and intestinal wall *(3)*. A ligature of 3-0 gut is grasped by the forceps, pulled through, and tied. This occludes one side of the vascular arcade. Note that the ligature *(4)* is being placed near a jejunal artery branch *(5)* that is not supplying the diseased portion of the bowel.

C   Both sides of the vascular arcade *(1)* have been ligated. The main jejunal artery *(2)* to the diseased bowel has been double ligated, and a branch from a second jejunal artery *(3)* next to the diseased bowel has been ligated.

100

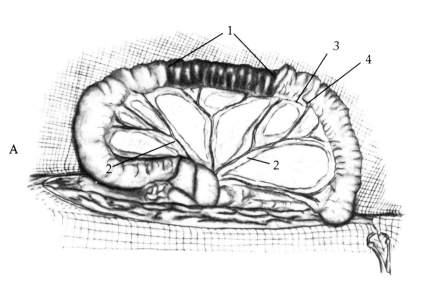

A

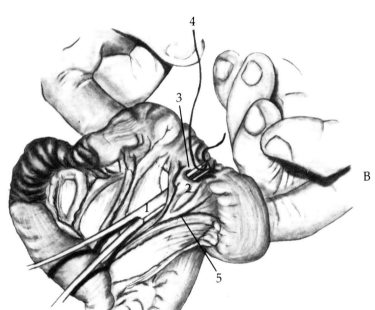

B

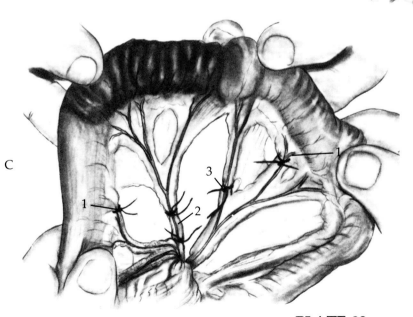

C

PLATE 32

Plate 33.   Two-layer resection and anastomosis

A   The mesentery has been incised to the intestinal wall. Note that the mesentery has been incised on the diseased side of the arcade ligatures *(1)*. This allows the ligature to remain with viable bowel and will prevent bleeding from the vascular arcade. A Carmalt forceps *(2)* has been applied to the intestine so that the tip of the forceps is on the diseased side of the arcade ligatures, leaving just enough space so a scalpel can be placed between the ligature and the Carmalt forceps. The handles of the forceps are placed at a 45-degree angle to the healthy side of the bowel *(3)*.

B   Noncrushing intestinal forceps *(1)* have been placed 3 cm away from the Carmalt forceps on the healthy bowel. The forceps may be rubber shod if the surgeon desires or not used at all. Some surgeons prefer to have an assistant occlude the bowel digitally. The bowel is being cut on the healthy side of the Carmalt forceps with a scalpel *(2)*. This incision should be smoothly and evenly made so that the cut edges of the bowel are left even. The resected bowel is discarded, and the remaining ends of the bowel apposed.

C   A 5-0 nonabsorbable suture with a swaged noncutting needle is used for the mucosal suture. The first suture stitch is placed midway between the mesenteric and amesenteric sides of the bowel. The suture is started by placing the needle through the submucosa and mucosa 2 mm from the cut edge of the left side *(1)* and then through the mucosa and submucosa of the right side *(2)*.

A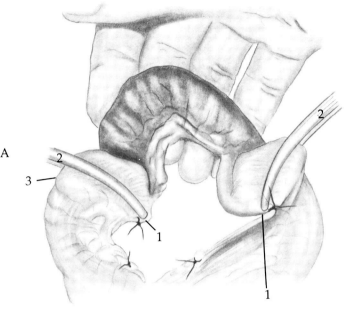

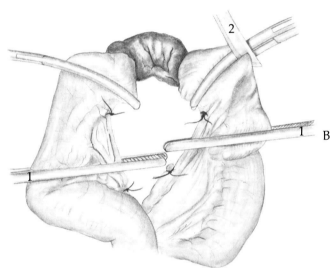 B

C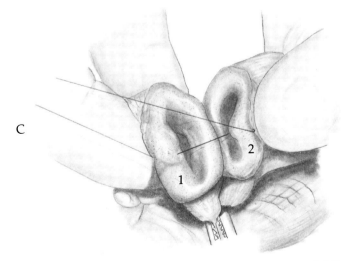

PLATE 33

103

Plate 34. Two-layer resection and anastomosis

A   The suture is tied, with the loose end being left long *(1)*. The remaining mucosa is apposed with a simple continuous suture pattern including the submucosa and mucosa *(2)*. The suture is carried toward the mesentric border of the intestine. As the mesenteric border is approached, the intestine is rotated 180 degrees by moving the handles of the intestinal forceps from right to left. The suture is continued to the site of the first stitch *(3)*. The last two to three loops of suture *(4)* are not tightened, allowing visualization for placement of the final stitches. The final stitch emerges at the knot *(5)* produced when the suture pattern was started. The loose loops of suture are individually tightened. The suture is tied to the loose end *(6)*, completing the mucosal suture pattern. It is important that a firm, even tension be maintained while the continuous suture is being placed. If such tension is not maintained, the mucosal apposition will not be tight. The mucosal suture line is tested for leaks by injecting sterile saline solution into the bowel lumen *(7)*. If any areas of leakage are present, these may be repaired with simple interrupted sutures. During placement of the mucosal suture pattern, the edges of the bowel should be handled gently. Very fine thumb forceps should be used, and the mucosa grasped 0.5 cm away from the cut edge. After the seal of the mucosal suture line has been demonstrated to be watertight, the intestinal clamps are removed. Note how the muscularis and the serosa are everted *(8)*.

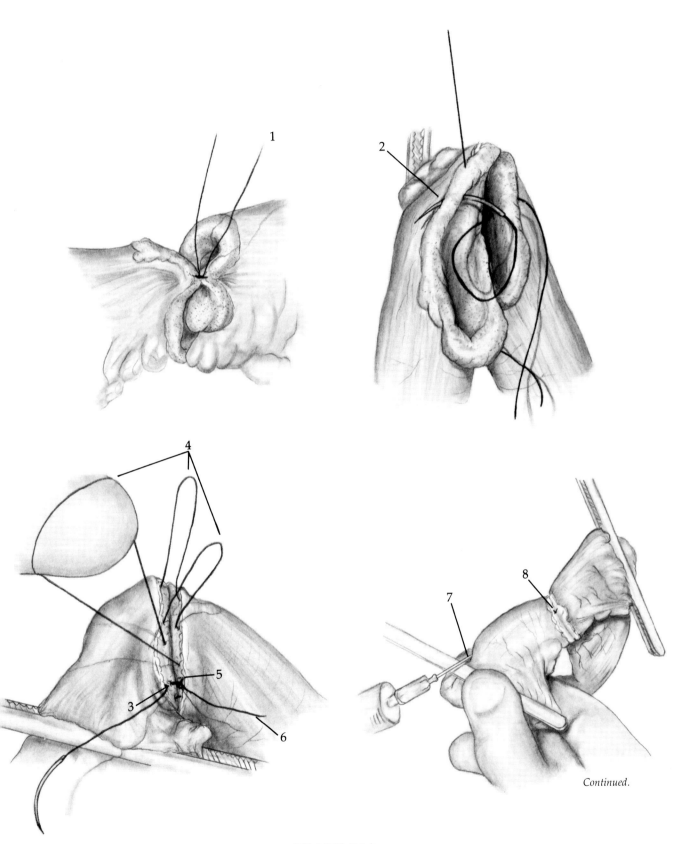

Continued.

PLATE 34A

Plate 34.   Two-layer resection and anastomosis—cont'd

B   The second row of sutures uses a Halsted pattern of 3-0 absorbable suture with a swaged noncutting needle to obtain serosa-to-serosa apposition. This suture penetrates the serosa and muscularis and picks up the submucosa. The stitch should be placed as close to the cut edge of the bowel as possible. The further from the edge the suture is placed, the more inversion of tissue occurs. The suture is started midway between the mesenteric and amesenteric borders of the intestine. The needle *(1)* is inserted down to the submucosa and out again next to the cut edge of the bowel *(2)*. The bite of tissue should be no more than 2 mm. The second stitch is placed on the opposite side of the bowel and is started next to the cut edge *(3)* and emerges *(4)* 2 mm away from the cut edge. The needle is reversed and inserted on the same side of the bowel in the same way—2 mm from the initial stitch *(5)*. The needle is carried to the other side, and the stitch *(6)* is placed 2 mm from the initial stitch. Note the reflection of mesentery *(7)* from the intestinal wall. This defect was created by spreading the forceps when the initial arcade ligature was placed, and it allows the mesenteric border of the intestine to be visualized while the sutures are being placed.

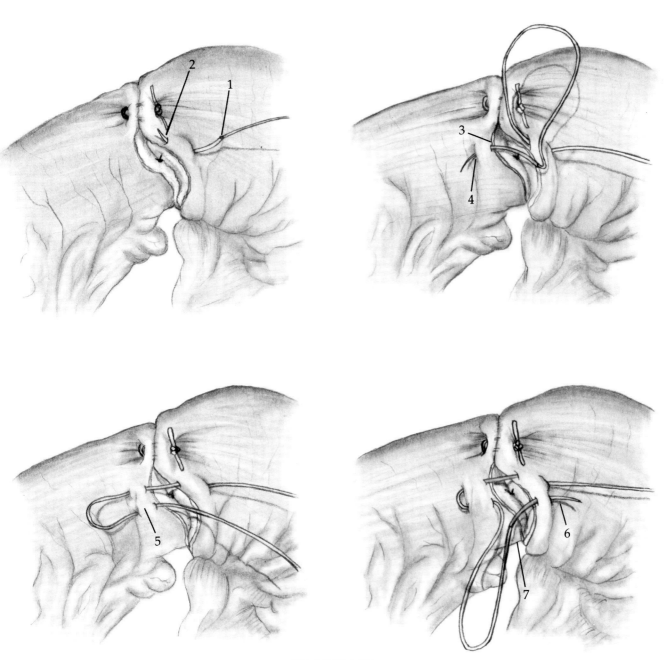

PLATE 34B

107

Plate 35.   Two-layer resection and anastomosis

A   A hemostat has been placed under the suture *(1)* as it crosses the incision. Downward pressure is placed on the hemostat as the suture is tied *(2)*. This produces inversion of the mucosa and allows for serosa-to-serosa apposition. The sutures are carried around the mesenteric border. If the dog is obese, the surgeon may find it easier to preplace the mesenteric sutures. This will allow complete visualization of the area. The Halsted sutures when completed should produce complete inversion of the mucosal suture line *(3)*. The mesentery is closed with a simple continuous 3-0 gut suture. Care must be taken when placing these sutures not to damage the jejunal arteries supplying the anastomoses. This two-layer suture pattern may be used to anastomose bowels of different diameters. This is often necessary when the anterior segment of bowel has dilated as a result of obstruction or when an intussusception involving ileum and colon has occurred. The bowel is prepared for anastomosis as described in Plates 32, *B*, to 33, *B*.

B   The lumen of the colon *(1)* is on the left, and the jejunal lumen *(2)* is on the right. Note the difference in size of the two lumens. The jejunal or smaller lumen is being incised *(3)* on the amesenteric border with scissors. The length of the incision should be as long as the difference in diameter size. When incised and opened, the smaller lumen should be the same diameter as the larger lumen. The two flaps *(4)* produced by the incision make up for the larger diameter of the opposite lumen. The first layer of sutures is begun at the bottom of the **V** *(5)* produced by the incision of the bowel. The suture is placed through the submucosa and mucosa. The suture is carried across the opposite lumen as in Plate 33, *C*, and tied as in Plate 34, *A*. This suture should be placed at the antimesenteric border of the larger lumen *(6)*. The remainder of the continuous suture is placed as described in Plate 34, *A*.

If too long an incision was made in the smaller bowel and it appears as if the bowel edges will overlap, placing the sutures closer together on the jejunal lumen and further apart on the colonic lumen will compensate for this. The final stitch of the continuous suture should emerge alongside the initial knot as described in Plate 34, *A*. The Halsted suture is placed as described in Plates 34, *B*, and 35, *A*.

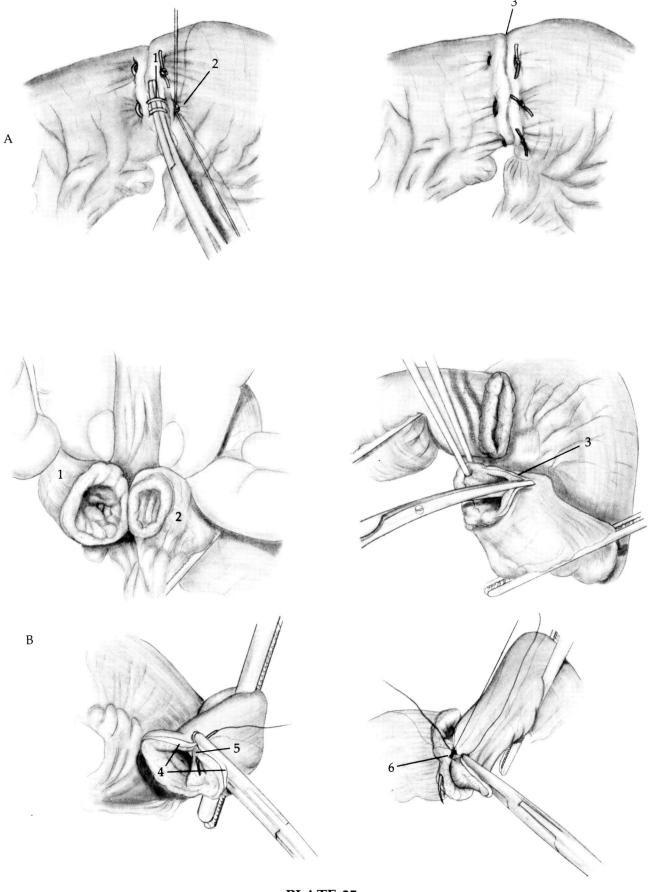

PLATE 35

Plate 36.   Resection and anastomosis with a Gambee suture

A   A schematic diagram of the Gambee suture pattern demonstrates the placement of the suture through the bowel wall. Note that the far bite *(1)* of the suture penetrates the full thickness of the bowel wall, whereas the near bite *(2)* penetrates only the mucosal layer. When the Gambee suture is tied, the mucosa is apposed, and at the same time a small amount of seromuscular inversion is produced.

B   The ends of the bowel have been apposed. The suture pattern is begun midway between the antimesenteric and mesenteric sides of the bowel. Three sutures have been placed. The needle *(1)* with swaged absorbable suture is inserted the full thickness of the bowel wall 3 mm from the cut edge *(2)*. The needle penetrates the left side from outside to inside.

C   The needle is reversed and penetrates first the mucosa *(1)* and then the submucosa *(2)* from inside to outside. Note that the seromuscular layer *(3)* is not included in this suture.

D   The submucosa *(1)* and mucosa *(2)* of the right side of the anastomosis is penetrated from outside to inside. Note again that the seromuscular layer *(3)* is not penetrated.

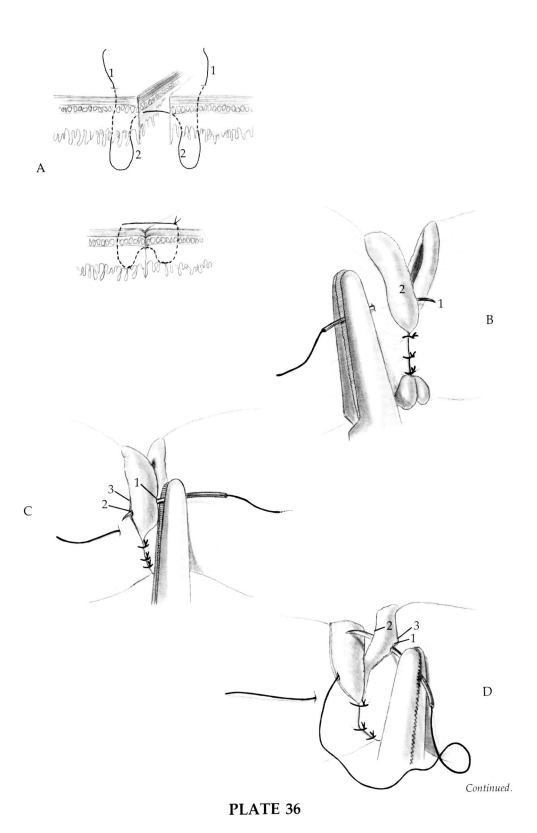

A

B

C

D

Continued.

PLATE 36

Plate 36.   Resection and anastomosis with a Gambee suture—cont'd

E   The needle is reversed, and the full thickness of the bowel wall is penetrated from inside to outside *(1)*.

F   The sutures are tied, producing a slight degree of serosal inversion. The suture pattern is carried around the bowel from antimesenteric side to mesenteric side. The last two or three sutures are preplaced.

G   The Gambee suture may also be used to produce end-to-end apposition of bowel of different-sized lumens. The antimesenteric side of the smaller diameter bowel segment is incised as described in Plate 35, *B*. The suture pattern is started at the **V** *(1)* made by the incision and carried to the antimesenteric border of the larger diameter bowel *(2)*. The second suture is placed from the flap *(3)* created by the small bowel incision to the larger lumen bowel. The anastomosis is completed as described in Plate 36. If the incision in the narrow segment was too long, the defect may be compensated for by placing the sutures further apart on the redundant side of the anastomosis and closer together on the smaller side of the anastomosis. The closure is completed as described in Plate 35. After completion of any intestinal anastomosis, the mesenteric defect should be repaired as described earlier.

The incision is checked for leaks by injecting sterile saline into the bowel lumen. If any leaks are present, they are closed with an interrupted Lembert suture.

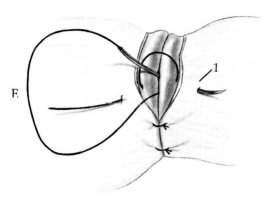

E

1

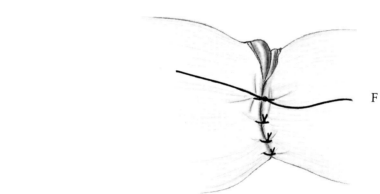

F

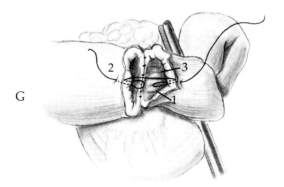

G

1

2

3

PLATE 36, cont'd

Plate 37. Resection and anastomosis with a crushing suture

A The bowel has been prepared as described in Plates 32, *B*, to 33, *B*. The ends of the bowel have been apposed. The anastomosis will be accomplished by a simple interrupted crushing technique. The needle *(1)* is passed through the full thickness of the wall 3 mm from the cut edge of the bowel.

B The needle *(1)* is passed on the opposite side from the inside of the lumen to the outside of the bowel wall.

C The first throw of the suture is tightened until the surgeon feels it cut through the mucosa and seromuscular layer. The suture is then tied. Note in the schematic drawing that the suture material has cut through the seromuscular layer *(1)* and mucosa *(2)*. The submucosa *(3)* is the tissue that the suture remains in. The suture is essentially buried if properly placed.

D Sutures are placed 2 to 3 mm apart. When tied, the sutures have a tendency to evert the mucosa slightly *(1)*. Note that the suture line is watertight immediately after finishing the repair.

Absorbable or nonabsorbable monofilament 3-0 suture may be utilized for this procedure.

If the surgeon desires, a second layer of Halsted sutures may be placed over the crushing sutures.

The techniques for apposing two different-sized lumens with a simple interrupted pattern are the same as described in Plate 35, only a simple interrupted suture is used.

The anastomotic site is thoroughly rinsed with a sterile saline solution, covered with omentum, and returned to the abdomen. The surgeon and assistant change gloves, gowns, and instruments, and the patient is redraped before the incision is closed.

If abdominal contamination occurred, the abdomen should be thoroughly rinsed with sterile saline solution and a lavage tube placed before the incision is closed (Chapter 8). The abdomen is closed (Chapter 8).

The postoperative dietary regimen is the same as that for enterotomy (Chapter 12).

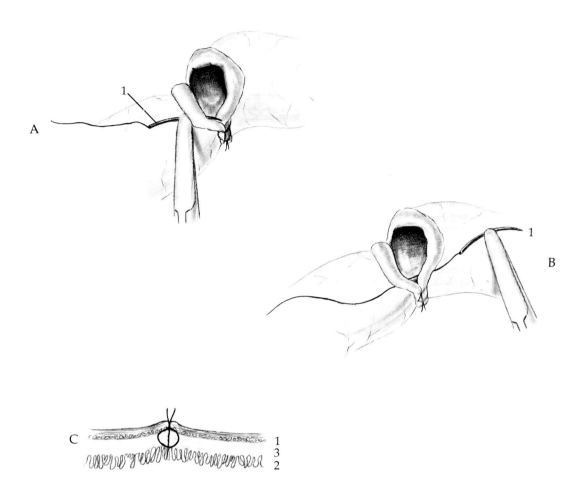

A

B

C

1
3
2

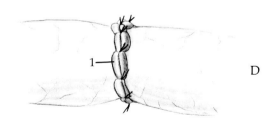

1

D

PLATE 37

115

GASTROINTESTINAL SURGERY

There have been many suture patterns described for closing hollow viscera following surgical manipulation. These may be divided into three main categories:

1. Inverting as demonstrated by the Connell-Cushing or Lembert-Czerny suture pattern
2. End-to-end apposition as demonstrated by the simple interrupted crushing suture pattern
3. A combination end-to-end/inverting effect as demonstrated by the two-layer mucosal Halsted suture or the Gambee suture patterns

In addition, these suture patterns may all be utilized to anastomose the intestine. This may be done with end-to-end, end-to-side, or side-to-side anastomotic techniques. Today most bowel anastomoses are performed with an open end-to-end surgical technique.

The reader is referred to the references for discussion of the merits of each of the various methods of hollow viscus closure. In this text an inverting suture pattern has been described for closing the stomach, and an end-to-end simple interrupted crushing suture has been described as one method for performing an intestinal anastomosis.

The other two suture patterns described for hollow viscus closure are a combination of the end-to-end and inverting techniques. One utilizes a simple continuous suture through the mucosa and submucosa for the first layer and a fine Halsted suture for the second layer. The continuous suture produces end-to-end mucosal apposition without inverting any tissue. The Halsted suture produces serosa-to-serosa apposition with minimal tissue inversion. Therefore both mucosal and serosal fibrin seal is obtained in addition to two lines of suture in the submucosa. The Gambee suture pattern also produces end-to-end mucosal apposition, but at the same time produces less serosal inversion than a Halsted suture. The reader will note that the two-layer closure and Gambee closure both eliminate mucosal eversion.

The biggest disadvantage of these suture patterns is that they require more time and skill to insert than the end-to-end crushing suture.

The reader can make a choice as to which method is preferred. The basic principles and the necessary knowledge of the anatomy for closing any hollow viscus remain the same.

REFERENCES

Abramowitz, H. B., and Butcher, H. R.: Everting and inverting anastomoses, an experimental study of comparative safety, Am. J. Surg. **121**:52, 1971.

Archibald, J., editor: Canine surgery, Santa Barbara, Calif., 1965, American Veterinary Publications, Inc.

Bennett, R. R., and Zydeck, F. A.: A comparison of single layer suture pattern for intestinal anastomosis, J. Am. Vet. Med. Assoc. **157**:2075, 1970.

Hertzler, J. H., and Tuttle, W. M.: Experimental method for everting end-to-end anastomosis in the gastrointestinal tract, Arch. Surg. **65**:398, 1952.

Path, E. J., and Gold, D.: Intestinal anastomosis, a unique technique, Am. J. Surg. **116**:643, 1968.

Reinertson, E. L.: Comparison of three techniques for intestinal anastomosis in the equidae, J. Am. Vet. Med. Assoc. **169**:208, 1976.

14
Nephrotomy

The usual purpose of a nephrotomy is to remove stones from the renal pelvis. Before proceeding, however, an evaluation of renal function is made. If the kidney containing the stones is not functional, it should be determined whether the remaining kidney is functional, and if so, a nephrectomy of the diseased kidney should be performed (Chapter 15).

A midventral abdominal incision is utilized to permit examination of both kidneys as well as the ureters during surgery.

Plate 38. Nephrotomy

A A midventral abdominal incision has been performed. The viscera have been packed off, and the diseased kidney exposed (Chapter 8). Note the increased blood supply in the peritoneum overlying the kidney and the lumpy appearance of the kidney (1).

B The peritoneum has been stripped off the kidney and reflected to the hilus of the kidney (1). The ureter, covered with fatty connective tissue (2), has been isolated and identified by palpation. The vessels lie cranial to the ureter (3). Bleeders are controlled by clamping and ligation. The area of the renal pedicle is not cleaned as it would be for a nephrectomy, since this would destroy the lymphatics and autonomic nerves associated with the vessels.

C The kidney is on stretch, and a Satinsky forceps (1) has been applied to the renal artery and vein contained in the fatty connective tissue (2). Note that the ureter is not included in the clamp (3). Clamping the ureter even for a short period of time may do permanent damage, resulting in a stricture formation within the ureter. It is important that all the renal vessels be included in the clamp. If the left kidney is involved, care should be taken to occlude all the renal arteries (Chapter 15). After applying the vascular clamp, one must not twist or pull the clamp because this will tear the renal vessels. The renal vessel may be occluded for 25 minutes. The less time of vascular occlusion, the better for the kidney.

D The kidney has been packed off and incised longitudinally along its lateral border. The incision, extending through the renal pelvis, should be made smoothly and evenly. Note the lack of hemorrhage. The kidney is opened, exposing the stone (1). The stone is removed and the pelvis examined to make sure all the stones have been removed. The ureter is palpated where it enters the hilus of the kidney to be sure that it is clear of stones.

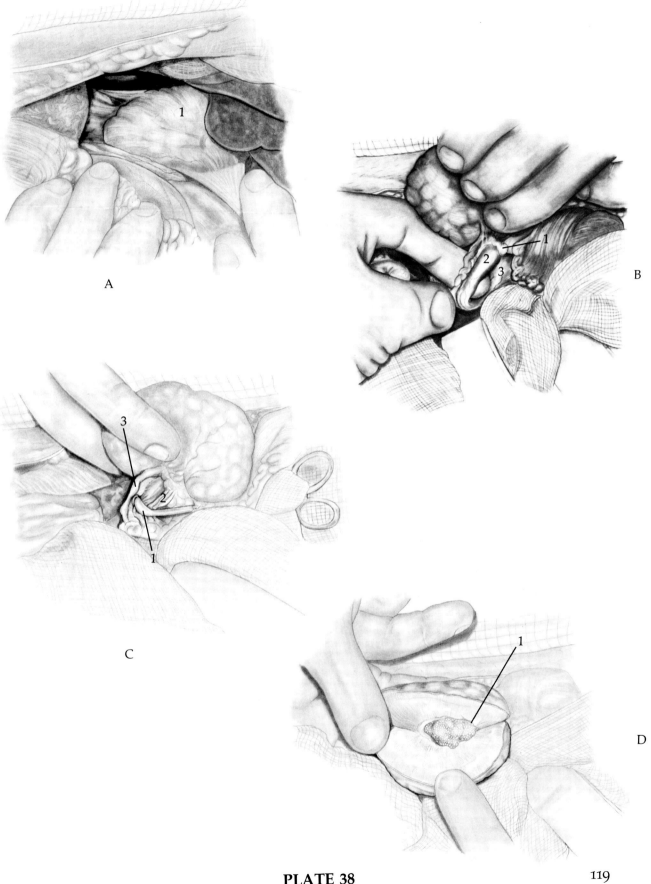

A

B

C

D

PLATE 38

Plate 39. Nephrotomy

A   The renal parenchyma is apposed and sutured with 0 medium chromic gut in a mattress suture pattern *(1)*. These sutures penetrate the capsule and parenchyma with a through-and-through pattern. They are placed about one fourth of the distance from the lateral border of the kidney and about 1 cm apart.

B   The mattress sutures have been placed and tied. Note that they appose the renal parenchyma. However, the edges of the incision gape open *(1)*. If the mattress sutures through the renal parenchyma are tied too tightly, this will increase the gapping of the incised edges. If left open, this incision will bleed when the blood supply is restored.

C   The edges of the renal incision are closed with a continuous interlocking suture of 2-0 chromic gut. The needle is passed through the renal capsule *(1)* and renal parenchyma *(2)* and tied. The suture pattern is continued by passing the needle *(3)* through the tissue and under the loop produced by the immediately preceding suture *(4)*. The suture pattern is continued to the end of the incision and tied to itself *(5)*.

D   This suture pattern should be evenly placed and tightened to appose the incision edges. Too much tension on the suture line will cut the renal tissue. It is important that each individual stitch be tightened as it is placed so that even tension occurs along the line.

The vascular clamp is removed, and the kidney is returned to the abdomen. Small tags of peritoneum may be pulled over the kidney to fix it in its normal position. The peritoneum does not have to be completely repaired. The abdomen is closed (Chapter 8).

The patient's renal function is closely observed and supported as necessary during the postoperative period.

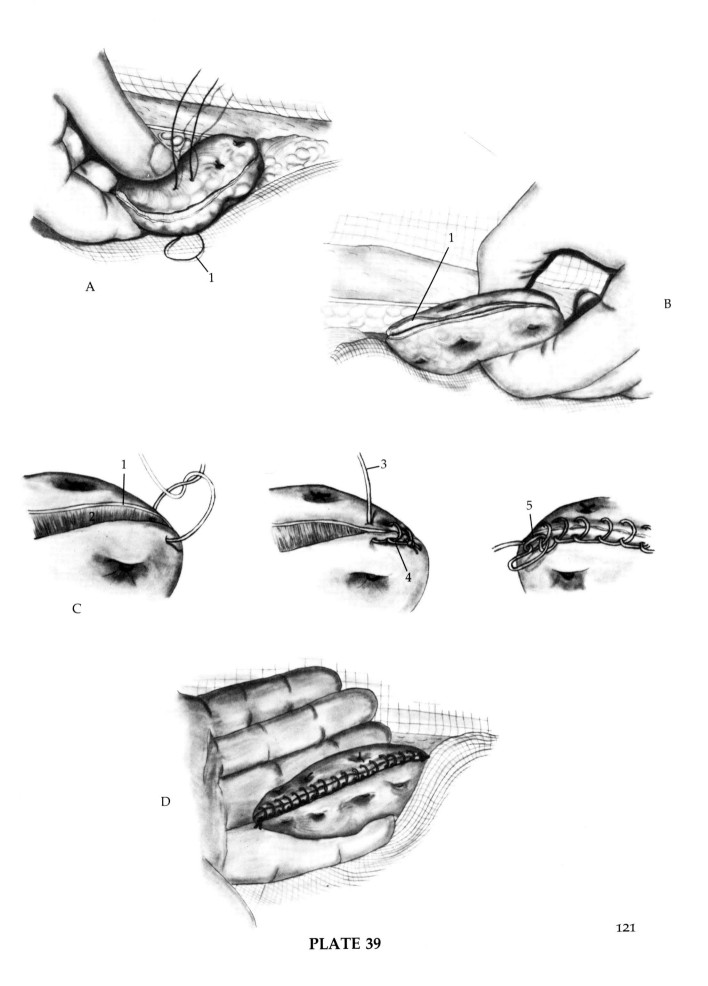

A

B

C

D

PLATE 39

15
Nephrectomy

Nephrectomy is performed to remove a diseased or nonfunctional kidney. The ability of the remaining kidney to function adequately should always be evaluated before such surgery is carried out. Most commonly nephrectomy is done to remove a hydronephrotic or pyelonephrotic kidney, but if a kidney contains renal calculi and is nonfunctional, it should also be removed.

Either of two approaches may be utilized. The flank approach permits nephrectomy without entering the peritoneal cavity; however, it makes examination of the opposite kidney difficult, if not impossible. The approach described here uses a midventral abdominal incision, which gives adequate exposure and permits examination of the entire urinary tract during the surgery.

Plate 40. Nephrectomy

A A midventral abdominal incision has been made. The abdominal viscera have been packed to the left side of the abdomen with a saline-soaked towel. A rib retractor *(1)* is spreading the abdominal incision for better exposure. The kidney is being elevated from the abdominal cavity. Note the vascular tissue overlying the kidney *(2)* and the fatty tissue around the renal pedicle *(3)*. This is the peritoneum under which the kidney lies.

B The peritoneum has been bluntly separated from the kidney and medial aspect of the renal pedicle, exposing the ureter *(1)*, the renal vein *(2)*, and the renal artery *(3)*. Note the remaining fatty tissue at the lateral aspect of the renal vessels *(4)*.

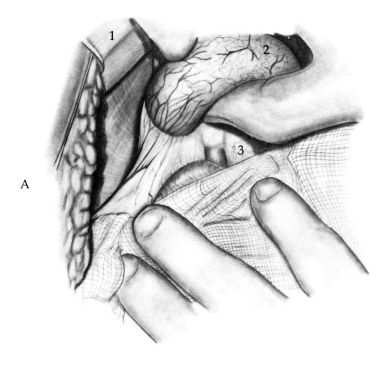

A

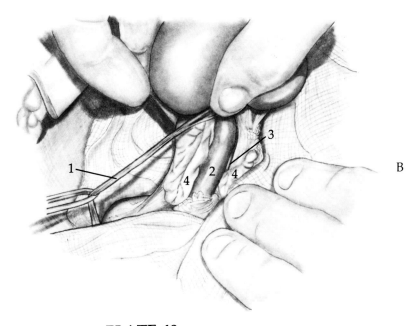

B

PLATE 40

125

Plate 41. Nephrectomy

A   The renal vessels have been completely cleaned of connective tissue. The kidney is on stretch, which elevates the caudal vena cava *(1)*. The surgeon must take care in removing the connective tissue not to damage the renal vessels, aorta, or caudal vena cava. It should be remembered that the left kidney will often have two and sometimes three renal arteries. It is therefore important that the pedicle be cleaned, so that when multiple arteries do exist, they can all be ligated. Note how the renal vessels branch before entering the hilus of the kidney *(2)*. For this reason it is important that the renal vessels be occluded close to their origin; otherwise a branch or a second renal artery may not be ligated, resulting in severe hemorrhage. Bleeders should be clamped and ligated so that the operative site is clearly seen. When dissecting the renal pedicle, the surgeon must take care not to damage the adrenal glands, which are located cranial to the kidney.

B   A double ligature of nonabsorbable material is placed on the renal artery close to where it arises from the aorta *(1)*. A single ligature is generally all that is necessary on the renal vein *(2)*. At the discretion of the surgeon, the arterial ligatures may be placed by transfixing the renal artery. Some surgeons prefer to mass ligate the renal pedicle, using a transfixing type of ligature. A clamp *(3)* is placed above the ligatures, and the renal artery and vein are divided between the ligature and clamp. During the entire operation, care should be taken when handling the diseased kidney. If the kidney is distended with fluid or pus, excessive pressure may cause it to rupture, resulting in abdominal contamination. If this occurs, peritoneal lavage should be done during closure (Chapter 8).

C   The ureter is double ligated and divided to finish the removal of the kidney.

The abdomen is closed, and appropriate antibiotics are used if needed. The patient's renal function should be closely observed during the postoperative period, and any necessary fluid and drug therapy instituted.

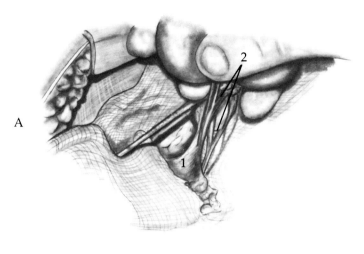

A

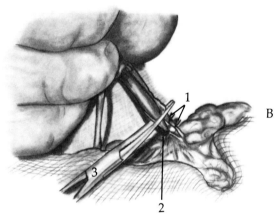

B

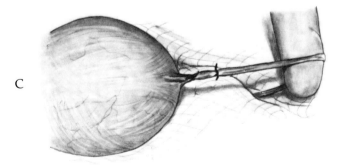

C

PLATE 41

127

16
Cystotomy

The primary indications for cystotomy are removal of cystic calculi, diagnosis of neoplasia, and evaluation of mucosal defects. Of these, the most common indication for surgery is cystic calculi.

After the incision site has been prepared, a sterile catheter is inserted, and as much urine as possible is removed. This sample should be cultured, and antibiotic sensitivity determined. If the urethra is obstructed, a urethrotomy may be necessary (Chapter 22).

A caudal ventral abdominal incision is made. The caudal abdomen is explored. Both kidneys and ureters should be examined by visualization and palpation. The prostate gland should be examined in the male. If neoplasia is suspected, the internal inguinal lymph nodes should be examined. If they are enlarged or feel abnormal, a biopsy is done.

Plate 42.   Cystotomy

A   The bladder is exposed, exteriorized, and packed off. This is accomplished by elevating its cranial end and reflecting it caudally. The initial incision is made in the least vascular part of the dorsal or ventral fundic area of the bladder. The length of the incision varies with the procedure. The incision should be long enough to remove all calculi and permit thorough examination of the interior of the bladder. Incision into the trigone area is generally not necessary to remove cystic calculi. However, when looking for an unknown source of bleeding or neoplasia, it may be necessary to examine this area. Care should be taken when incising the region of the trigone not to damage the ureteral orifices. The incision should be placed midway between them. To prevent ureteral damage, proper positioning of the bladder when exteriorized is important. If the bladder is twisted, damage to one of the ureteral openings could occur, either by incision or by occlusion after closure of the bladder.

B   The calculi have been removed from the bladder. Now the bladder should be digitally palpated, especially in the area of the trigone. In the male dog a sterile catheter should be passed to be sure no calculi are left in the urethra. In the bitch the catheter is passed from the bladder into the vagina. The inner surface of the bladder should be examined for ulcers or polyps after removal of the calculi. If ulcers are present, they may be treated by silver nitrate cautery. Occasionally an ulcer will have eroded a small vessel, producing hemorrhage. This small bleeder may be ligated, or silver nitrate cautery may be used to stop the bleeding. If polyps are present, a biopsy should be done. If generalized neoplasia is identified, the degree of involvement of the bladder and the extent of metastasis will determine the course to be followed. If cystic calculi or chronic infection is present, the bladder wall will be thick, and the mucosa (1) will be thickened, hemorrhagic, and friable. Therefore the Allis tissue forceps (2) should be applied only if necessary to obtain exposure and then only for a very short period. Stay sutures may be used for traction instead of tissue forceps. If sutures are used, they should not penetrate the lumen.

After exploration of the bladder and just prior to closure, the bladder may be flushed with sterile saline solution to remove sand and clots. A culture should be taken of the bladder mucosa prior to flushing.

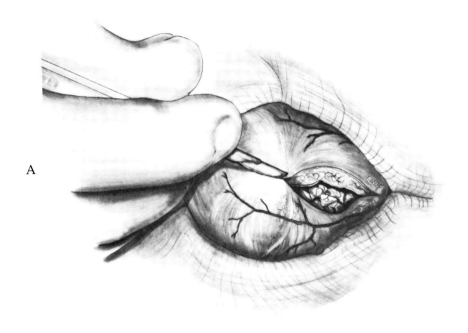

A

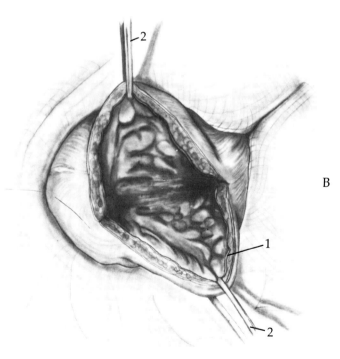

B

PLATE 42

131

Plate 43. Cystotomy

A   The bladder is closed with a two-layer suture pattern, using 3-0 absorbable suture with a swaged noncutting needle. The first layer is placed in the submucosa, without penetrating the mucosa. This apposes the mucosa with a watertight seal but does not introduce any foreign material into the lumen of the bladder to act as a nidus for subsequent calculi formation. The suture pattern is begun at one corner of the incision. This suture should be started just past the end of the mucosal incision. It is inserted parallel to the incision and mucosa on the far side (1). Allis tissue forceps may be gently used to retract the serosa and muscularis.

B   The needle is reversed, and the near side is sutured in the same manner as the far side.

C   Note the position of the suture. When the knot is tied, the mucosa and the submucosa will be apposed.

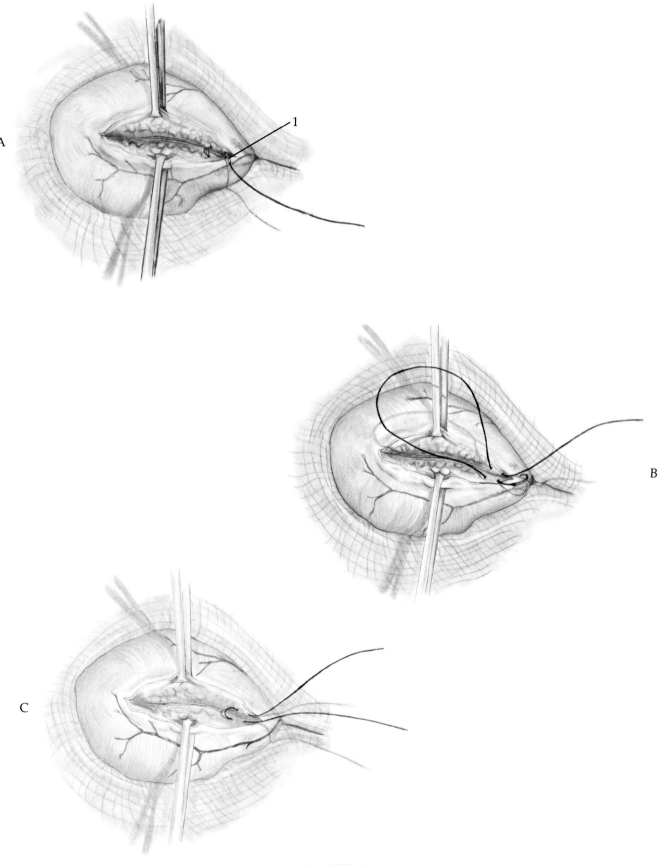

PLATE 43

Plate 44.   Cystotomy

A   The second suture *(1)* is placed through the submucosa at the opposite end of the incision.

B and C   Note the way the placement of the sutures is altered. The incision is sutured from both ends toward the middle.

D   The final suture has been placed *(1)*. The surgeon will generally find it easier to preplace the last two or three sutures. This allows visualization for placement of the final suture.

E   The first suture layer is finished *(1)*. Note that the sutures do not overlap. After all the first-layers sutures have been tied, the bladder may be checked for leaks by filling it with sterile saline solution. If a small leak should be present, the opening may be closed with a simple interrupted suture in the submucosa. The second suture layer apposes the seromuscular layer. These are simple interrupted sutures of 3-0 absorbable suture *(2)*. They are placed through the serosa and muscularis and pick up some of the submucosa.

After closure of the second layer, the bladder surface is flushed, the bladder is returned to the abdomen, and the drapes are removed. The surgeon and assistant surgeon then change gloves, gowns, and instruments before closing the abdomen. The abdomen is lavaged with povidone-iodine (Betadine) solution (Chapter 8).

Postoperatively, appropriate drug therapy should be instituted.

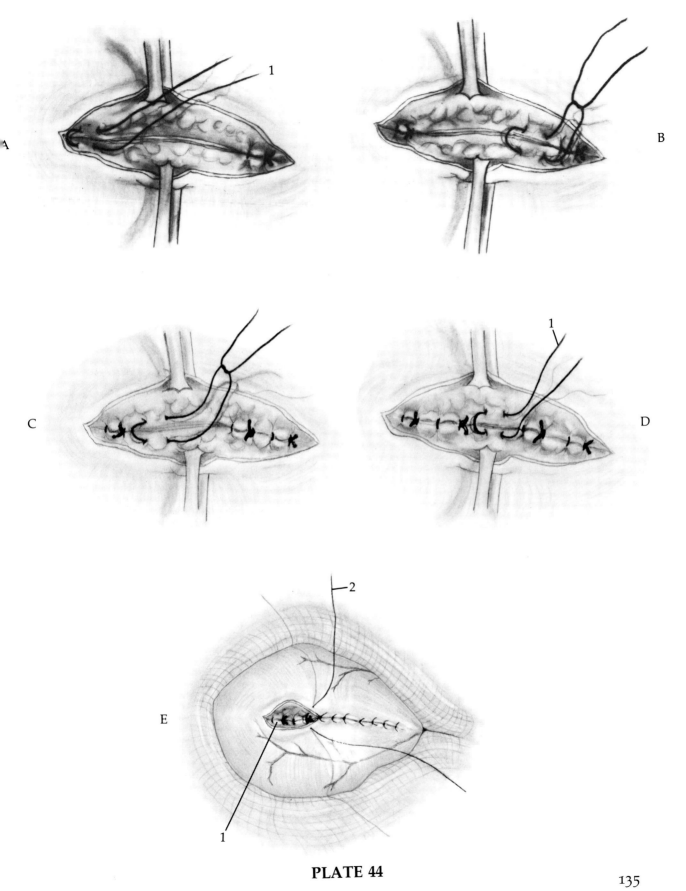

A

B

C

D

E

1

1

2

1

1

PLATE 44

135

REFERENCES

Finco, D. R.: Current status of canine urolithiasis, J. Am. Vet. Med. Assoc. **158**:327, 1971.

Leonard, E. P.: Fundamentals of small animal surgery, Philadelphia, 1968, W. B. Saunders Co.

17
Ovariohysterectomy for pyometritis

Pyometritis is usually a disease of older bitches. Generally these patients are toxic and, consequently, require careful preoperative and postoperative attention.

The surgical technique used for removal of a pus-filled uterus is similar to any standard ovariohysterectomy technique. The main variation is to oversew the uterus to prevent spillage of pus with resultant contamination of the abdominal cavity. This same technique may be used for ovariohysterectomy when the uterus is enlarged, for example, in metritis or a postpartum uterus.

Plate 45. Ovariohysterectomy

A A caudal ventral midline incision is made (Chapter 7). Since the uterus may be distended, care must be taken when entering the abdomen not to damage the uterus. The uterus is gently exteriorized because it usually is friable when distended and may rupture easily. Therefore an adequate initial abdominal incision must be made so that the uterus can be exteriorized easily without excessive handling or pulling on this distended organ. Note the fatty broad ligament *(1)* and the distribution of the uterine artery and vein alongside the body of the uterus *(2)*.

B Either ovary may be grasped with the thumb and index finger and tension applied in a ventral and caudal direction. The suspensory ligament of the ovary *(1)* may then be palpated as it runs from the ventral aspect of the ovary *(1)* to its dorsal attachment at the middle and ventral third of the last ribs. The ovarian vessels *(2)* are located caudal to the suspensory ligament. In the obese bitch the ovarian artery and vein are not easily visualized. Caudal ventral traction on the ovary relaxes the artery and vein, preventing damage to them when the ligament is broken or severed. It is important that the ovary be oriented normally when traction is applied. If the ovary should be reversed, the ovarian artery and vein could be damaged when the suspensory ligament is severed. While one hand is applying traction to the ovary, the index finger of the opposite hand is placed where the suspensory ligament is attached *(3)*, and the ligament is strummed as if it were a guitar string until the ligament is broken. In some cases, where the attachment is strong, the suspensory ligament may be severed with scissors just below its ovarian attachment.

C The broad ligament is spread, and the ovarian artery and vein *(1)* identified. A small hole is made caudal to the ovarian artery and vein by putting a closed Carmalt forceps through the broad ligament. Note the loop of bowel *(2)* behind the broad ligament.

D Three Carmalt forceps are placed beneath the ovary, including the ovarian vessels and fatty tissue. The ovarian stump is divided between the top two Carmalt forceps. The top forcep, which is attached to the ovarian side of the stump, is reflected caudally. The reflected broad ligament may be clamped with the Carmalt forceps anterior to the uterine vessels and mass ligated to control potential bleeders. This is necessary in the obese bitch or in the bitch with a post-partum uterus.

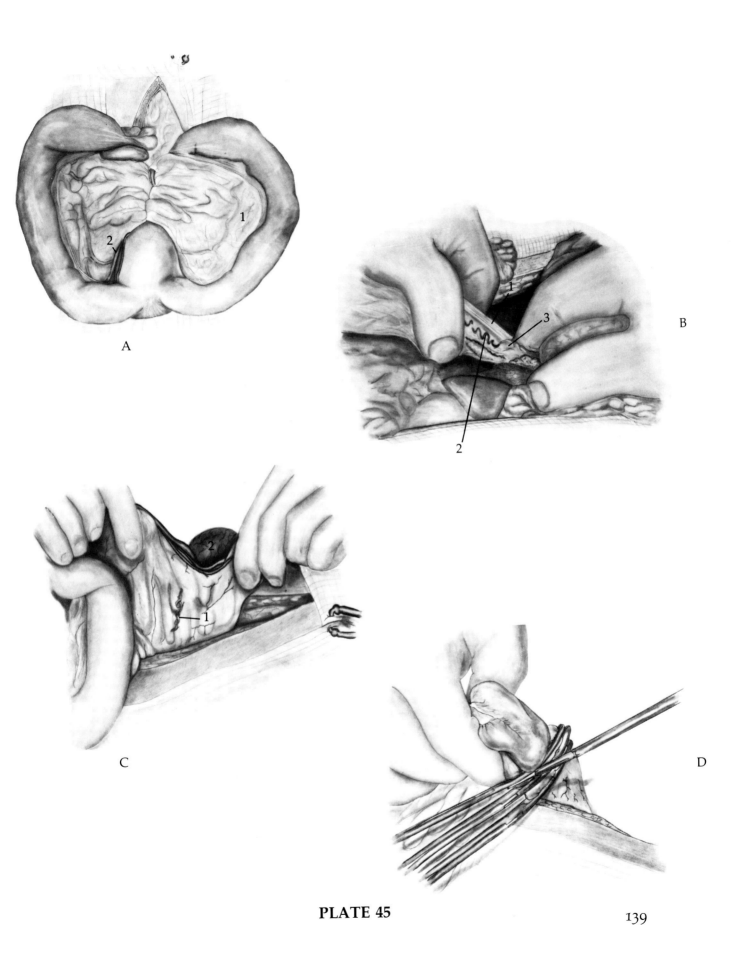

PLATE 45

Plate 46. Ovariohysterectomy

A   The first ligature is placed below both of the remaining Carmalt forceps. When the ovarian stump is large because of excessive fatty tissue, a fixation ligature is recommended. If the stump is small, mass ligation works satisfactorily. To place the fixation ligature, a hemostat *(1)* is passed through the ovarian stump. The absorbable ligature material is grasped by the hemostat and pulled through the stump.

B   The first tie is made on the cranial aspect of the ovarian stump with a surgeon's knot.

C   The long end of the ligature *(1)* is passed completely around the ovarian stump and is again tied with a surgeon's knot.

D   The lowest Carmalt forceps is removed, and a second mass ligature is placed in the area crushed by the Carmalt forceps. This mass ligature is tied with a surgeon's knot.

E   The ovarian stump is grasped with a hemostat, and the last Carmalt forceps removed. The two ligatures are observed for tightness and leakage. The ovarian stump is gently placed into the abdominal cavity and is closely observed for signs of bleeding. If the stump is dry, it is released. It is important that the ovarian stump be examined after the tension has been released, since tension on the ovarian vessels will often prevent hemorrhage. Moreover, the ligatures may appear tight while the stump is under tension but may slip after the tension is released. The second ovary is removed with the same technique.

If the ovarian stump and vessels should break or slip away while being manipulated, fatal hemorrhage can result. To recover the ovarian vessels, the surgeon should extend the incision 2 to 3 cm cranial to the umbilicus and lower the dog's head, thus removing most of the viscera into the cranial abdomen. If the right vessels have been dropped, the mesoduodenum is used to pack the viscera to the left aspect of the abdomen. If the left vessels have been dropped, the mesocolon is used to pack the viscera to the right aspect of the abdomen (Chapter 8). The packing of the viscera will expose the kidney. By examining the area at the caudal pole of the kidney, the ovarian vessels can be located. Gentle traction on the broad ligament will help identify the vessels. Since the ureters are in close apposition to the ovarian vessels, the surgeon must not ligate or blindly clamp this area until sure that the ureters are not included in the tissue.

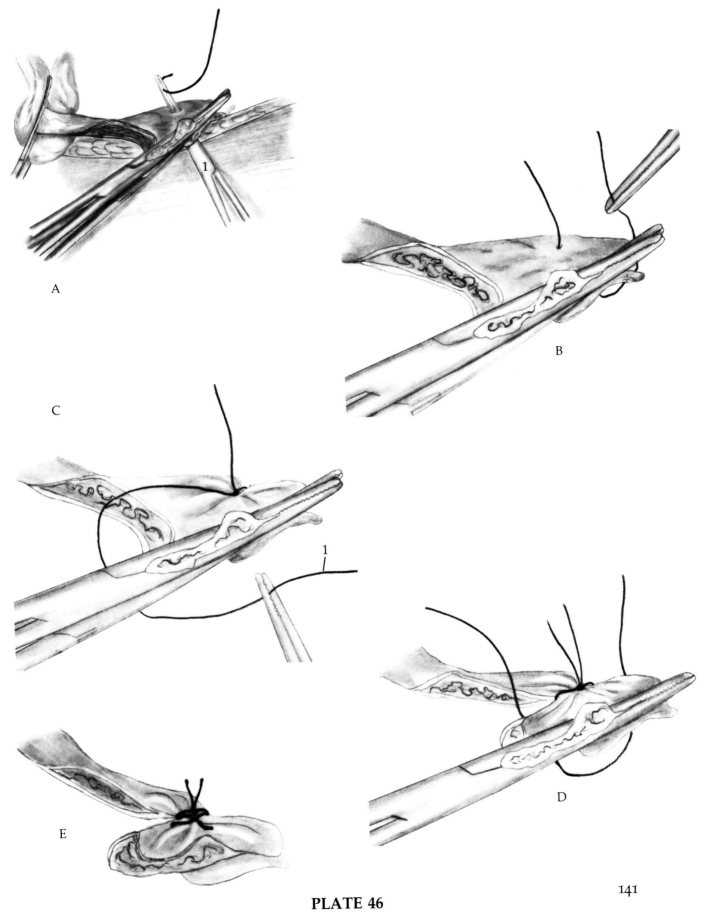

A

B

C

1

D

E

PLATE 46

141

Plate 47. Ovariohysterectomy

A   Traction is placed on the uterine horns so that the body of the uterus is exteriorized. The uterine vessels are identified lateral to the uterine body. A hemostat is passed between the uterine vessels and the body of the uterus (1) just proximal to the cervix. The absorbable ligature material is grasped with the hemostat and pulled around the vessel. The vessel is ligated with a surgeon's knot on each side.

B   Two Carmalt forceps are placed just proximal to the ligatures (1) across the uterine body. The uterine body is divided between these forceps. The uterus and ovaries are discarded. If the uterus is infected, the cut end of the stump may be cauterized with a silver nitrate stick or a 2% iodine solution on a swab.

C   A Cushing suture pattern is loosely placed over the Carmalt forceps on the uterine stump. This suture pattern is similar to a Connell suture (Chapter 10), except that it does not penetrate the mucosa. The needle is inserted through the seromuscular layer and submucosa at one edge of the uterine body parallel to the Carmalt forceps (1). The needle is advanced and placed on the opposite side of the Carmalt forceps (2). This pattern is continued until the uterine stump and Carmalt forceps have been oversewn. The final suture emerges from the uterine body (3). The initial suture and final suture should be placed to prevent penetration of the uterine vessels below the ligature (4).

D   The Carmalt forceps is gently opened and withdrawn. At the same time, traction is placed on both ends of the suture, causing the edges of the uterine stump to invert.

E   The two ends of the Cushing suture are tied, thus exerting a pursing effect on the uterine stump. The uterine stump is gently placed in the abdomen and examined for bleeding. If it is dry, the suture is cut. A second Cushing suture may be placed over the first layer in lieu of tieing the two ends together.

If the uterine artery or stump is dropped, the incision should be extended caudally to the pubis. The urinary bladder is grasped and exteriorized. The uterine stump will be seen on the dorsal aspect of the urethra just caudal to the neck of the bladder. When recovering a dropped uterine artery or stump, care should be taken not to clamp or ligate the urethra or the ureters, which are located at the trigone of the bladder. Excessive traction on the bladder can damage the ureters.

After closure of the uterine stump, the abdomen is closed. If the uterus was infected, appropriate systemic antibiotics should be given.

If the uterus ruptured during or prior to surgery, the technique of peritoneal lavage described in Chapter 8 may be used to treat or prevent peritonitis.

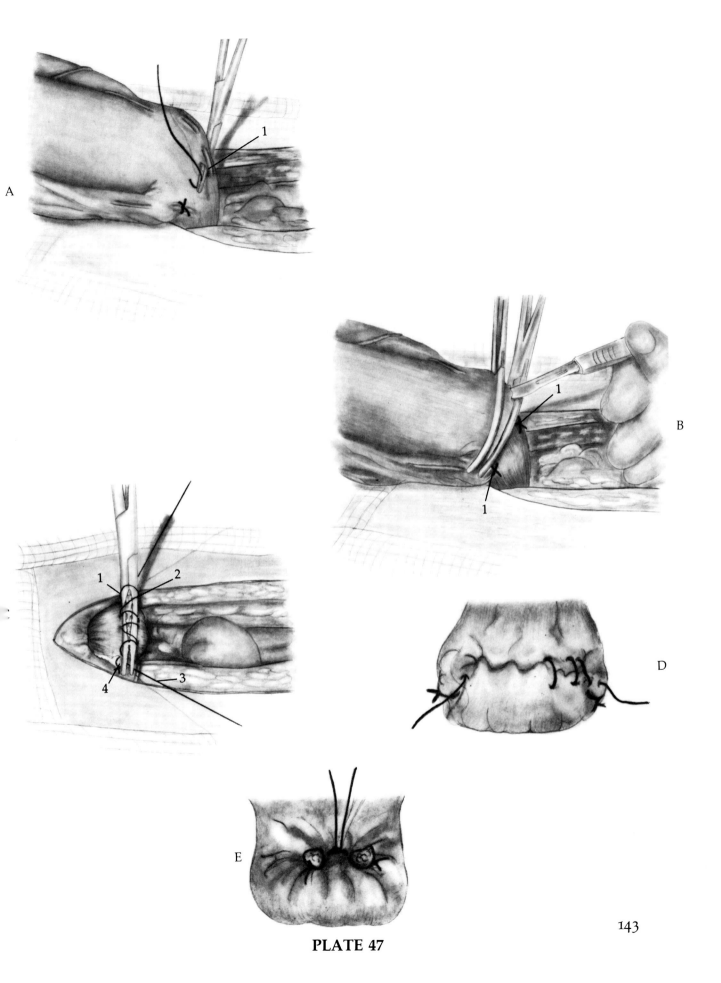

A

B

C

1
2
4
3

D

E

143

PLATE 47

18
Aortic embolectomy

Aortic embolectomy is presented to demonstrate a method of invading the aorta to remove a clot. The basic technique may be applied to any larger vessel. The suture pattern may be used to close any vascular defect.

The surgeon should remember that removing the clot from a vessel does not eliminate the cause of the clot. Unless the disease process causing the clot is identified and treated, reccurrence of the clot is not uncommon.

There appears to be in the stagnated blood in the hind legs an elevation of potassium that could be high enough to produce cardiac arrhythmias, fibrillation, or arrest when this blood reaches the heart. After the vessel is repaired, the sudden return of blood flushes out the stagnated blood with its elevated potassium content, which could result in the death of the animal. To prevent this the blood flow to the occluded area should be returned gradually, and calcium should be available to counteract the potassium effect.

Plate 48.   Aortic embolectomy

A   The abdomen has been opened with a ventral midline abdominal incision. The viscera are packed into the cranial abdomen with a saline-soaked towel. The peritoneum and fatty tissue have been dissected off the aorta *(1)* and vena cava *(2)*. This tissue should be completely removed from all aspects of the aorta. The aorta must be completely free above and below the site of the clot. This is necessary to cross clamp the aorta. The external iliacs *(3)* and internal iliacs *(4)* must also be mobilized. Also, it is usually necessary to ligate and divide the lumbar arteries. The number of lumbar arteries divided depends on the size of the clot and how far cranially the aorta needs to be mobilized. The deep circumflex iliac arteries *(5)* have also been divided. It is better not to ligate these vessels unless necessary to obtain mobility of the aorta. Bleeders in the tissue dissected free from the aorta are controlled by clamping and ligation. It is important to control hemorrhage to maintain good visibility of the surgical site. All connective tissue must be completely removed from the area of the anticipated aortic incision *(6)*. If this area is not clean, difficulty will be experienced when repairing the incision.

B   The aorta is mobilized. A straight patent ductus clamp *(1)* has been placed across the aorta, occluding it. The aorta has been incised over the clot *(2)*. The clot can be seen extruding from the incision. The caudal mesenteric artery is cranial to the clamp. If the clot were larger, this vessel would have been isolated and occluded with a bulldog clamp.

C   The clot has been removed, and a 3½ French polyethylene catheter *(1)* has been passed into the external iliac artery *(2)*. Immediately after removing the clot and before passing the catheter, the surgeon should examine the iliac vessels for bleed back. The presence of bleed back indicates that the vessels are patent. The catheter is passed as far as possible, and the vessel is flushed with heparinized saline solution. The remaining iliac arteries are flushed in the same manner. After the vessels are flushed, it is generally necessary to occlude the iliac vessels with a second patent ductus clamp to control bleed back and to maintain a clear surgical site.

D   The aorta has been closed in a two-layer crisscross simple interrupted suture pattern with 5-0 cardiovascular suture with a swaged needle (Chapter 4).

The caudal occluding clamp is removed first to allow bleed back. The cranial clamp is removed 5 minutes after the caudal clamp is removed. This clamp should be removed slowly over a 15- to 20-minute period. Cardiac function should be closely observed during this time.

If any leaks in the suture line occur, they should be closed with a simple interrupted suture of 5-0 silk. The abdomen is closed routinely (Chapter 8).

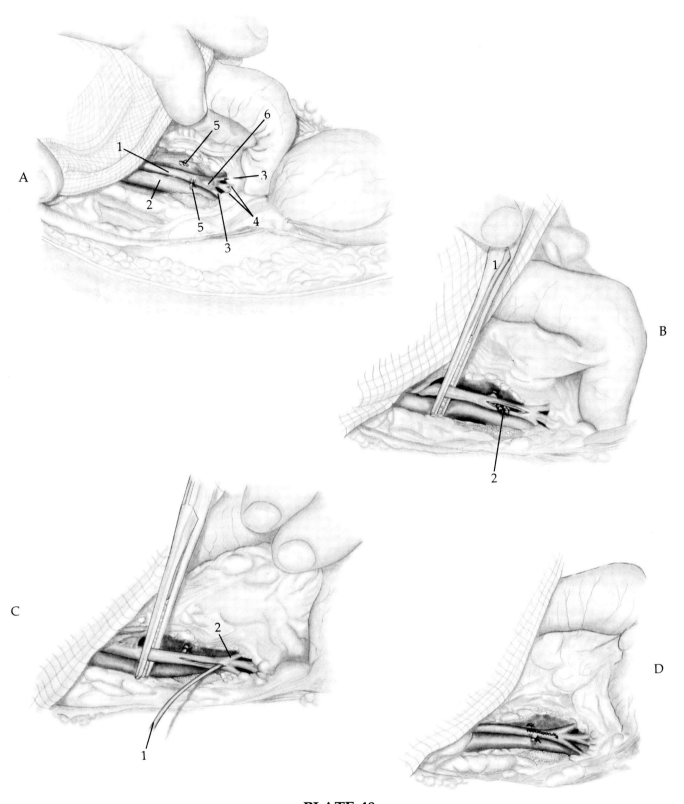

PLATE 48

REFERENCE

Freak, M. J.: Symposium on thrombosis. I. Arterial thrombosis embolism in the cat, J. Small Anim. Pract. 7:717, 1966.

PART FOUR
MISCELLANEOUS SOFT TISSUE

19
Modified Lacroix-Zepp ear drainage

The modified Lacroix-Zepp operation is often the treatment of choice for chronic otitis externa. The objects of the surgery are to expose the horizontal ear canal to the air so that it may dry and to promote drainage of exudates. Moreover, the cartilage flap acts as a drainboard to allow easier treatment of the ear and to reduce irritation from infective material draining from the ear.

The operation will improve a chronic ear infection, and if surgery is performed before severe granuloma formation or ossification of the cartilage occurs, it is generally curative.

If the ear is acutely infected, the acute infection should be brought under control before surgery is performed. This is accomplished by thorough cleansing of the ear, followed by antibiotic therapy based on culture of the ear.

If both ears are involved, the surgery may be done bilaterally during one anesthesia period.

Twelve hours prior to surgery the ears are filled with a cerumenolytic agent. After anesthesia has been induced, the surgical site clipped, and the ears thoroughly flushed with soap and water, the surgical scrub is performed. The ear is then filled with surgical antiseptic, and the animal is draped.

Plate 49. Modified Lacroix-Zepp procedure

A   The right ear is to be operated on, and the dog is placed in left lateral recumbency. The dotted line depicts the surgical incision site.

B   A grooved director (1) is inserted into the vertical ear canal and is advanced to the point where the vertical ear canal becomes horizontal. This is the point just below the tragus. The end of the groove director is palpated, and a horizontal skin incision is made about 0.5 to 1 cm below this level (2). This incision should be slightly shorter than the distance between the intertragic incisure (3) and the tragohelocine incisure (4). The horizontal incision is connected to the incisures to complete the skin incision. This skin incision should extend only through the skin and not include the subcutaneous tissue. The skin flap is grasped by Allis tissue forceps (5).

C   Traction is placed on the Allis tissue forceps, and with scissors the skin is dissected from the subcutaneous tissue. Bleeders are controlled by clamping and ligating. The skin flap now serves as a "handle" to manipulate the surgical area.

D   The subcutaneous tissue at the top of the ear canal is incised down to the cartilage (1). With scissors the subcutaneous tissue is reflected from the cranial, caudal, and lateral aspects of the vertical cartilage. This is best done bluntly, especially at the lower portion of the ear canal, to prevent damage to the parotid salivary gland. The parotid salivary gland lies partially on the auricular cartilage; therefore the tissue overlying the auricular cartilage should not be indiscriminately incised. Control of hemorrhage is essential to maintaining a clear field.

152

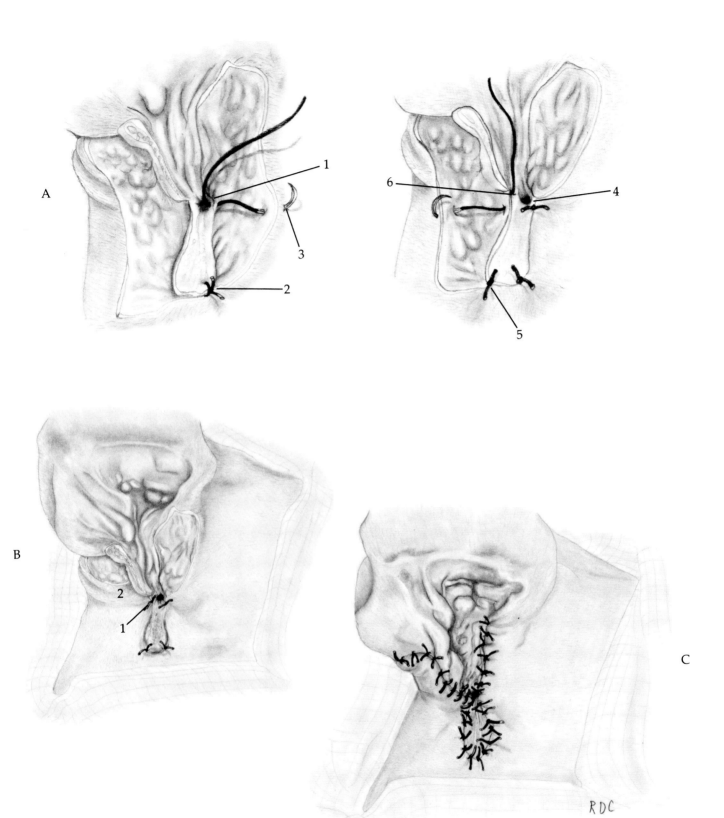

PLATE 51

REFERENCES

Fraser, G., Gregor, W. W., MacKenzie, C. P., Spreull, J. S. A., and Withers, A. R.: Canine ear disease, J. Small Anim. Pract. **10**:725, 1970.

Hoffer, R. E.: Otitis externa and media. In Kirk, R. L., editor: Current veterinary therapy, vol. VI, Philadelphia, 1977, W. B. Saunders Co.

20
Episioplasty

Perivulvular dermatitis is generally seen in the older obese bitch. In many cases the bitch has been spayed before puberty, resulting in an immature vulva. As the bitch ages and becomes obese, the vulva is surrounded and almost covered by redundant skin. In some bitches the vulva is almost obscured by this redundant skin. As the bitch urinates, the urine dribbles over the perivulvular skin, producing an irritation, especially in the deepened folds alongside and above the vulva. This chronically irritated skin becomes secondarily infected, resulting in perivulvular dermatitis. The problem is aggravated by a swelling secondary to the inflammation and irritation that makes the condition more difficult to treat.

Episioplasty removes the redundant skin and excess fat, thus exposing the vulva and eliminating the folds where the chronic irritation and inflammation occur. If possible, acute perivulvular infection should be treated and brought under control before any surgery is performed.

Plate 52.   Episioplasty

A   An Allis tissue forceps has been placed on the skin fold above the vulva. Traction is applied dorsally to expose the vulva and to estimate the amount of excess skin to be removed. Note the deep folds alongside the vulva *(1)* and above the vulva *(2)*. Also note how the vulva *(3)* is recessed in the depression formed by this excess skin.

B   The anus is closed with a purse-string suture prior to scrubbing and draping. The dog is placed in sternal recumbency, with the hind legs positioned over the end of the table. An Allis tissue forceps is placed on the vulva, and ventral traction is applied. The initial skin incision is made about 5 mm from the outer border of the vulva. The incision is started at the most ventral aspect of the vulva *(1)* and is carried dorsal to the vulva and down to the ventral aspect on the opposite side of the vulva *(2)*. There should be 5 mm of skin attached to the vulva when the incision is finished *(3)*.

C   The second incision is started at the base of the vulva *(1)*. This incision is carried dorsally and then ventrally to the ventral aspect of the first incision *(2)*. The distance between the two incisions is determined by the amount of excess skin to be removed. Note that the distance is narrower at the ventral aspect of the incision than at the dorsal aspect. The dorsal towel clamp is placed on the ventral aspect of the anus. The incision should not reach the anus. The skin between the two incisions is dissected free from the underlying subcutaneous tissue. If there is excess fatty tissue, this also may be removed by scissors. All bleeders are controlled with ligatures of 3-0 chromic gut.

If in doubt as to how much skin to remove, the surgeon should remove less than appears necessary. The closure should be evaluated as described in Plate 53, *A,* and if more skin needs to be removed, it should be done at that time rather than remove too much skin with the initial incisions.

160

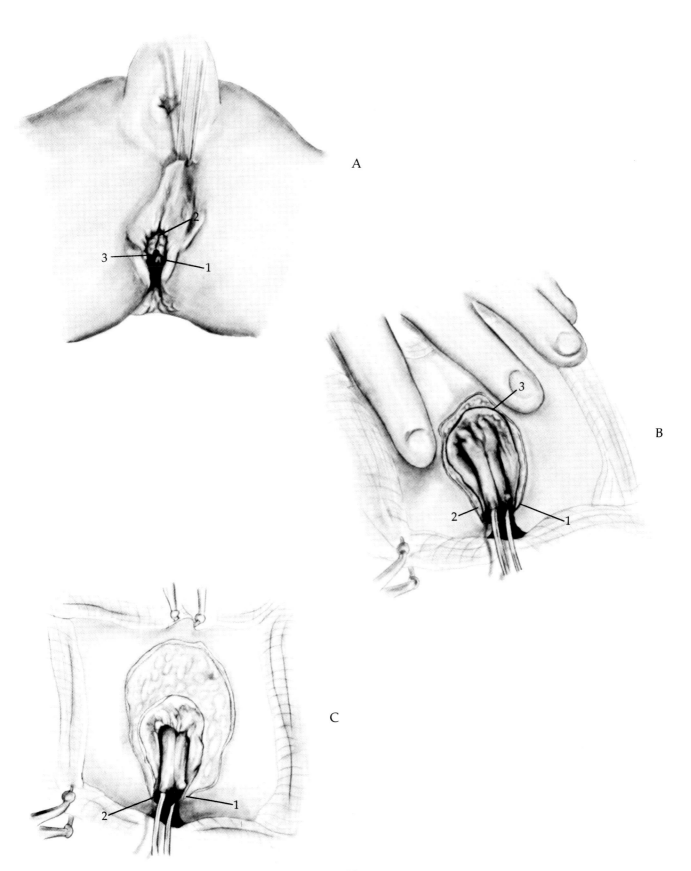

PLATE 52

Plate 53.   Episioplasty

A   A suture of nonabsorbable material is placed through the middle of the dorsal aspect of the vulvar flap *(1)* and directly on the midline of the perianal region *(2)*. This suture may be pulled tight before tying to evaluate whether enough skin has been removed. When this suture is tight, traction may be placed on the lateral aspects of the vulvar flap. This should completely expose the vulva and eliminate the deep folds that were present on the lateral aspects of the vulva. If this has not been accomplished, more skin should be removed from the outer incision. It should be emphasized at this point that all bleeding should be controlled in the subcutaneous area. Formation of a seroma predisposes to infection and poor healing of the surgical site. Also, excessive swelling in this area will cause the dog to lick at the sutures, with resultant breakdown of the wound.

B   The closure is completed with a simple interrupted suture pattern of nonabsorbable material. The second and third sutures are placed at 3 and 9 o'clock. The remainder of the incision is closed by placing a suture midway between 12 and 3 o'clock and between 12 and 9 o'clock and then midway between 3 and 5 o'clock and between 9 and 7 o'clock. The next sutures are placed midway between those previously placed. This technique is continued until the entire incision is completely closed.

Postoperatively, the purse-string suture is removed from the anus. Antibiotics are administered in accordance with the degree of contamination or infection present. The dog should be put in an Elizabethan collar to prevent mutilation of the incision. Alternate sutures may be removed 10 days postoperatively, and the remaining sutures, 14 days postoperatively.

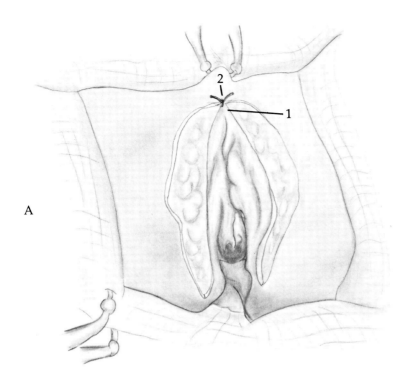

A

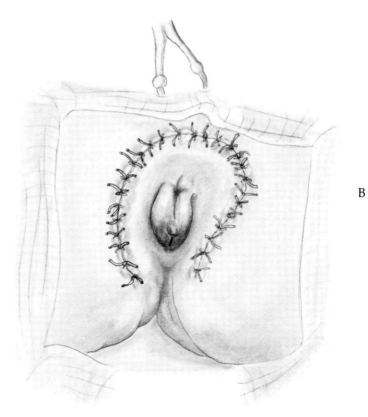

B

PLATE 53

21
Perineal urethrostomy

Perineal urethrostomy is performed in the male feline to eliminate the problem of recurrent urethral obstruction. The object of the surgery is to eliminate the narrow penile urethra, the site of most obstructions. The remaining wide pelvic urethra is sutured to perineal skin, and first-intention healing occurs. Therefore the chance of granulation tissue forming, with subsequent stricture, is reduced, and the wide urethral opening is maintained. In addition, the technique of Wilson and Harrison utilizes the penile urethra as a drainboard so that the incidence of irritation in the perineal region is minimized.

The animal is prepared for surgery and placed on the table in *dorsal* recumbency with the hind legs pulled forward, so in reading the description of the surgery, remember that the cat is on his back. A purse-string suture is placed in the anus before the surgical area is asepticized.

Plate 54. Perineal urethrostomy

A An elliptical incision has been made around the penis and scrotum. The incision should be about 3 to 4 mm ventral to the anus. This elliptical piece of skin, including the scrotum and prepuce, is dissected free. The dissection is begun at the dorsal aspect of the incision *(1)*. At this point the cat, if intact, should be castrated. Blood vessels supplying the penis, prepuce, and scrotum should be clamped and ligated.

B The penis *(1)* has been completely isolated and freed of connective tissue, and the attached skin and prepuce *(2)* are reflected ventrally and cranially. This isolation is accomplished by careful scissors dissection. Once the penis has been isolated, continued dissection will expose the ischiocavernous muscles *(3)*, which are usually covered with fat and should be carefully dissected free.

C The ischiocavernous muscles *(1)* have been isolated. Fatty tissue *(2)* is being reflected away with an Allis tissue forceps. The right muscle is isolated by retracting the penis to the left side. The cranial and caudal borders of the right muscle and root of the penis are completely exposed. A closed mosquito forceps is inserted beneath the muscle and root and carefully opened, thus freeing these structures. This forceps *(3)* is then withdrawn and clamped in the middle. The left muscle and root are isolated by retracting the penis to the right.

D The forceps is removed from the ischiocavernous muscle and root after 5 minutes, and they are severed with scissors *(1)*. Clamping effectively controls hemorrhage. All the muscle fibers and penile attachments must be severed to free the pelvic urethra. Cautery may be used when severing the muscle and root.

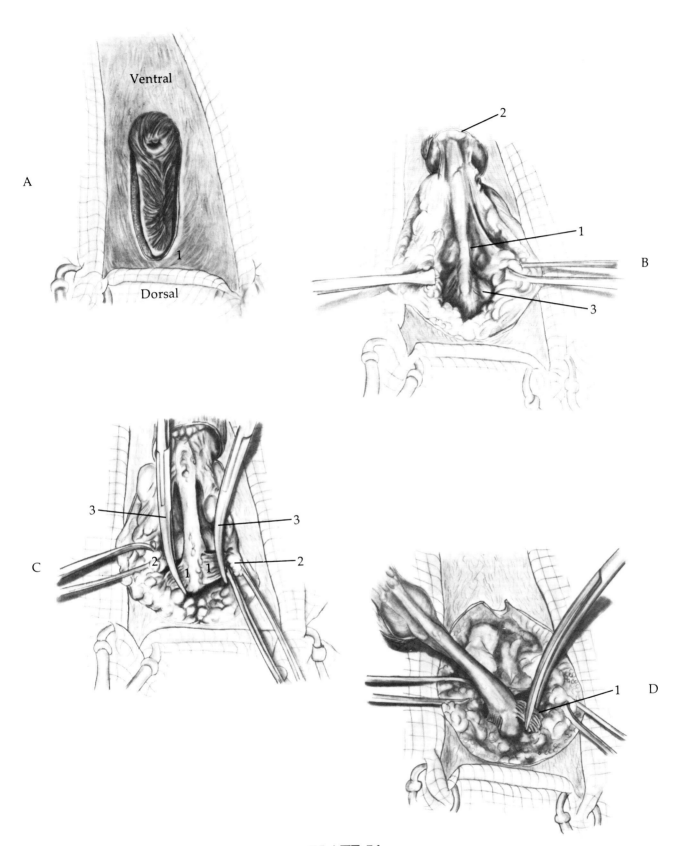

PLATE 54

Plate 55. Perineal urethrostomy

A The penis is being retracted in a caudal-dorsal direction to expose the connective tissue attachment *(1)* of the pelvic urethra to the symphysis pubis. This attachment is carefully incised with scissors *(2)*. Care must be taken not to cut the pelvic urethra. Note the incised ischiocavernous muscles *(3)*. After the ventral pelvic urethral attachments have been severed, the pelvic urethra can be completely mobilized by careful digital dissection.

B Traction is applied to the penis in a ventral-cranial direction. This traction is applied until the bulbourethral glands are well exposed *(1)*. If the bulbourethral glands cannot be visualized, either the ischiocavernous muscles or the ventral attachment of the pelvic urethra has not been completely separated. Note the purse-string anal suture *(2)*. The retractor penis muscle may be seen on the penis *(3)*. If it is not visible, further dissection of the loose tissue on the penile surface will expose it.

C A disposable sterile polyethylene tomcat catheter has been passed into the penile urethra and on into the bladder (Plate 55, D). The retractor penis muscle *(1)* has been grasped by thumb forceps and is being dissected free. This dissection is continued past the bulbourethral glands *(2)*, and the muscle is removed. Traction is maintained on the penis in a ventral direction during the dissection *(3)*.

D An incision *(1)* has been made into the penile urethra over the catheter. This initial incision may be made with a No. 11 Bard-Parker blade. Note the catheter in the penile urethra *(2)*.

168

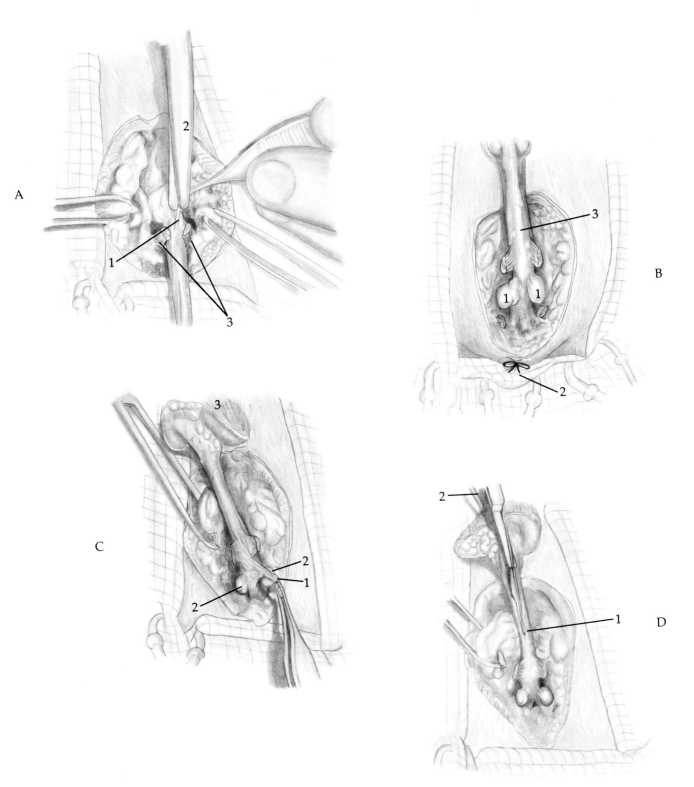

PLATE 55

Plate 56. Perineal urethrostomy

A After the urethra has been entered, the urethral incision (1) is extended with a small iris scissors toward the bulbourethral glands. This is accomplished by inserting the blunt blade alongside the catheter within the urethra.

B The urethral incision (1) is continued proximal to the bulbourethral glands (2). The urethral mucosa can be visualized (3). A fine thumb forceps is used to handle the urethra. Care must be taken not to damage the urethral mucosa. Note the tomcat catheter and the way traction separates the urethral wall from the urethral mucosa.

C The urethral mucosa is sutured to the skin using 5-0 nonabsorbable suture with a swaged needle. A preplaced simple interrupted suture pattern is utilized for the initial three sutures. The needle is passed through the urethral mucosa and skin at 6 o'clock (1). The second suture is placed at 7 o'clock (2). The third suture is placed at 5 o'clock (3). After these sutures have been placed, traction is put on them to see if they will evenly and totally appose the urethral mucosa to the skin edge (4). The area in which it is most important to obtain apposition is at the dorsal aspect of the incision (4). If this area is not properly apposed, the sutures should be repositioned. Note how the proper suture placement spreads the urethral orifice (5). The next two sutures (6,7) will continue to spread the urethral orifice. The two most important aspects of the suture technique are first to pick up the urethral mucosa only and appose it to the skin and second not to leave any defects at the union of the skin and mucosa. Occasionally, if the skin incision has been extended too far dorsally, it may be necessary to preplace the urethral sutures and then suture the skin defect at the dorsal aspect. The important point to remember here is not to narrow the urethral orifice.

D The remainder of the urethral mucosa is sutured to the perineal skin with a simple interrupted suture pattern for one-half to two-thirds the length of the penis. This will vary with the condition of the urethral mucosa. If there have been repeated obstructions or attempts to catheterize the cat, the more distal urethral mucosa will be damaged, necessitating its removal. A mattress suture is placed across the penis and tied proximal to where the penis will be amputated (1). This will control bleeding from the cavernous tissue. The penis is amputated below this suture. The skin is sutured to the end of the penis, and the remaining skin defect closed to itself with simple interrupted sutures (2). The purse-string suture is removed from the anus.

The animal is treated with appropriate medication for control of the cystitis. A protective ointment such as zinc oxide is applied to the surgical site for the first week. The sutures are removed at 10 to 14 days postoperatively.

During the first and second postoperative day, manual compression of the bladder two to three times a day may be necessary. The cat should be observed closely to make sure that excessive licking of the surgical site does not occur. If the cat licks at the surgical site, an Elizabethan collar may be used.

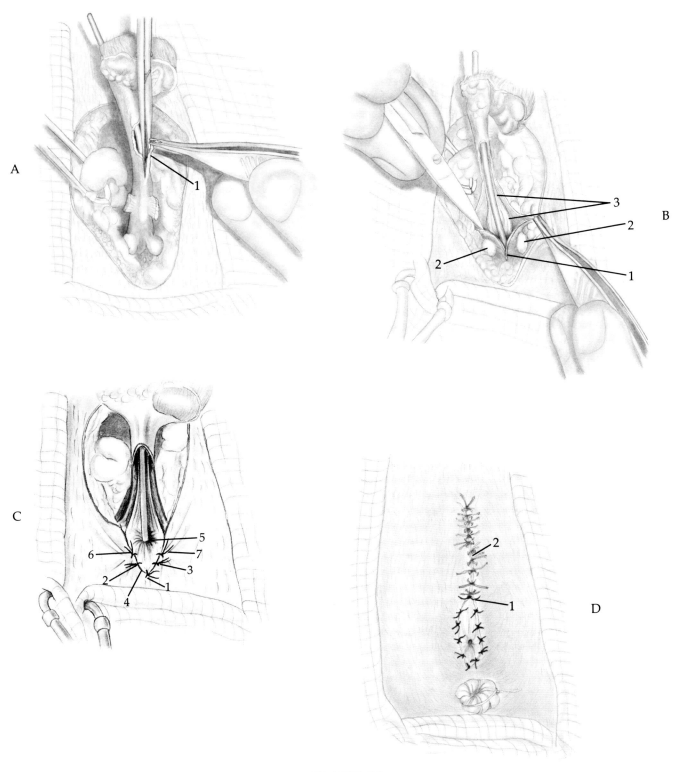

A

B

C

D

PLATE 56

REFERENCE

Wilson, G. P., III, and Harrison, J. W.: Perineal urethrostomy in cats, J. Am. Vet. Med. Assoc. **159**:1789, 1971.

22
Urethrotomy

In the male dog, urethral obstruction may occur from urinary calculi lodging behind the os penis, and occasionally behind the ischial arch. A dog with urethral calculi may also have cystic calculi; therefore it may be necessary to perform a cystotomy in conjunction with a urethrotomy. When a urethrotomy is performed as an emergency procedure in a dog that is toxic from prolonged obstruction, a cystotomy is then accomplished after the dog's condition has stabilized. When a urethrotomy is performed on a toxic patient, only a local anesthetic at the incision site need be used. Occasionally calculi may also be lodged at the brim of the pelvis, and these usually can be dislodged and removed through the urethrotomy incision. If they cannot be dislodged, a perineal urethrotomy may be necessary.

The area around the sheath and scrotum is clipped. The clipped area and the prepuce are thoroughly washed and antiseptic applied.

Plate 57. Urethrotomy

A   A sterile catheter is passed until the obstruction is reached. The tip of the catheter is palpated *(1)*, and the skin and subcutaneous tissue *(2)* over it are incised, exposing the penis *(3)*. If the stone is lodged within the os penis, the incision should extend from the caudal end of the os penis toward the scrotum. The skin incision should be at least 1 cm in length, but may be longer if necessary. The incision may be extended cranially over the os penis or caudally to the scrotum. Bleeders are controlled by clamping and ligation.

B   The urethra is opened over the end of the catheter by incising the retractor penis muscle, the corpus cavernosum urethrae, and the urethral mucosa as a unit *(1)*. Generally after these tissues have been incised, the pressure in the bladder resulting from the obstruction will force the proximal urethral calculi through the incision. If any calculi remain in the os penis, they are removed by mosquito hemostats and catheter manipulation. The catheter should be passed into the bladder to make sure the urethra is patent. Note that the penile incision is shorter than the skin and subcutaneous incision *(2)*. This will prevent urine from accumulating under the skin during the healing processes.

If the patient's condition is stable and calculi are in the bladder, a cystotomy is then performed, with separate drapes, instruments, gowns, and gloves being used (Chapter 16).

Healing occurs by second intention. Bleeding from the incision site generally persists for 3 to 4 days after surgery. Appropriate antibiotics are used systemically, and an ointment may be applied to the skin in the area of the incision to prevent irritation from urine scald.

A

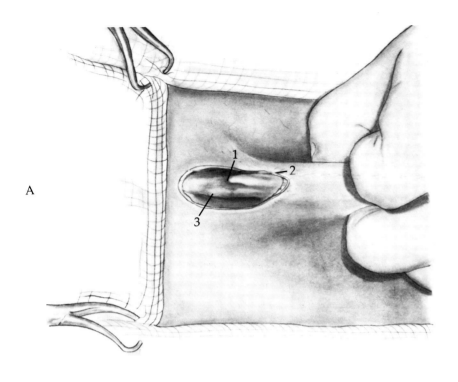

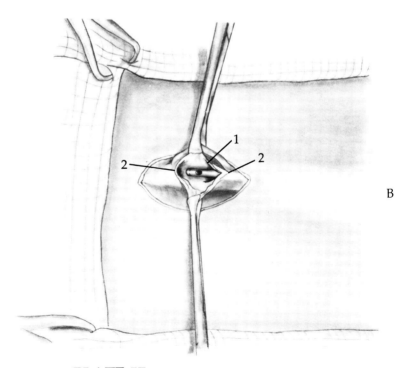

B

PLATE 57

175

23
Scrotal urethrostomy

A scrotal urethrostomy is performed when a permanent urethrostomy is necessary. This is usually done to treat chronic cystic calculi, especially ureate calculi. The procedure may also be used to maintain urethral patency in conjunction with penile amputation for neoplasia, severe trauma, or stricture formation.

The technique depends on accurate apposition between the urethral mucosa and the skin. Good apposition will produce primary healing without excess granulation and subsequent stricture.

The dog is placed on the table in a dorsal recumbent position. The skin and inside of the sheath should be thoroughly washed and prepped prior to sterile insertion of a urinary catheter.

Plate 58. Scrotal urethrostomy

A A skin incision is made around the scrotum. This incision must be planned to leave enough skin to suture to the urethral mucosa without excess tension. The initial incision may be made more conservatively, since more skin can be removed prior to urethral suture if necessary.

B The scrotum and testicles *(1)* are removed as a unit after ligation of the spermatic cord. This dissection will expose the penis *(2)*. Bleeders should be controlled by ligation.

C The retractor penis muscle *(1)* is dissected free and removed at the most caudal-dorsal *(2)* aspect of the incision.

D The urethra *(1)* is opened on the midline with a No. 15 Bard-Parker blade. The incision is extended to the point where the penis begins to bend dorsally *(2)* over the ischiatic arch.

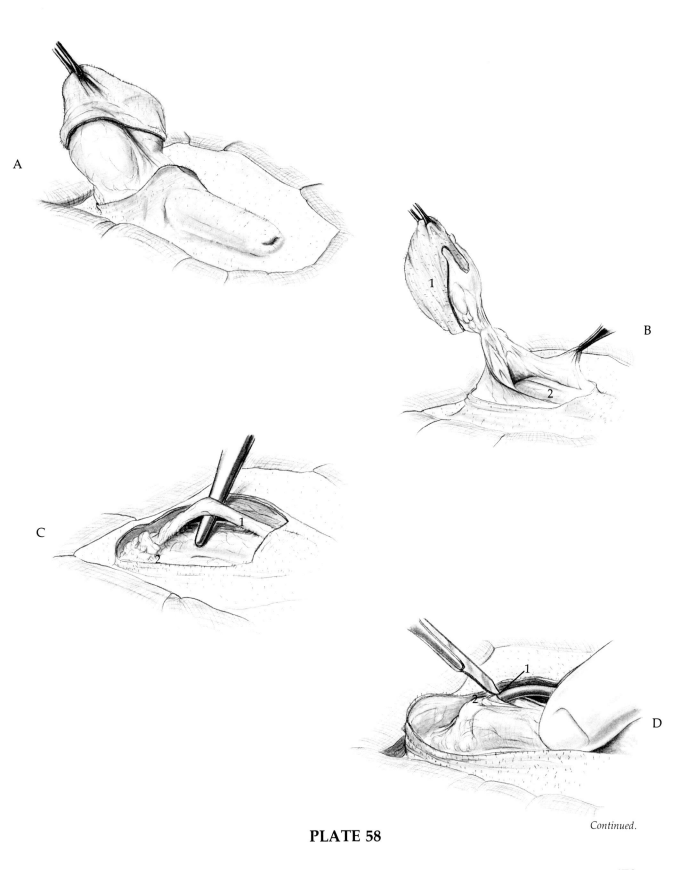

PLATE 58

Continued.

Plate 58. Scrotal uretheostomy—cont'd

E   The urethral mucosa *(1)* is sutured to the skin with fine nonabsorbable sutures using a simple interrupted pattern. The closure is started at the most cranial aspect of the urethral incision *(2)*. Note that the urethral mucosa and skin are in good apposition.

F   The cranial aspect of the skin incision *(1)* is closed. Sutures are placed on alternate sides of the incision, moving caudally. Note the mucosal/skin apposition at the cranial portion of the incision *(1)*. Note also the position of the catheter in the caudal portion of the urethral incision.

G   The most dorsal aspect of the urethral incision is sutured to the skin *(1)*, and the skin dorsal to the incision *(2)* is closed. It is important to obtain accurate apposition of the urethral mucosa to the skin. This will reduce the amount of bleeding in the postoperative period.

Bleeding from the operative site will occur for 5 to 7 postoperative days. This bleeding will be minimal unless the suture line breaks down.

The dog should be prevented from licking the site. Protective soothing ointments may be applied to the site. Systemic antibiotics should be utilized. Sutures should be removed in 10 days if healing is satisfactory.

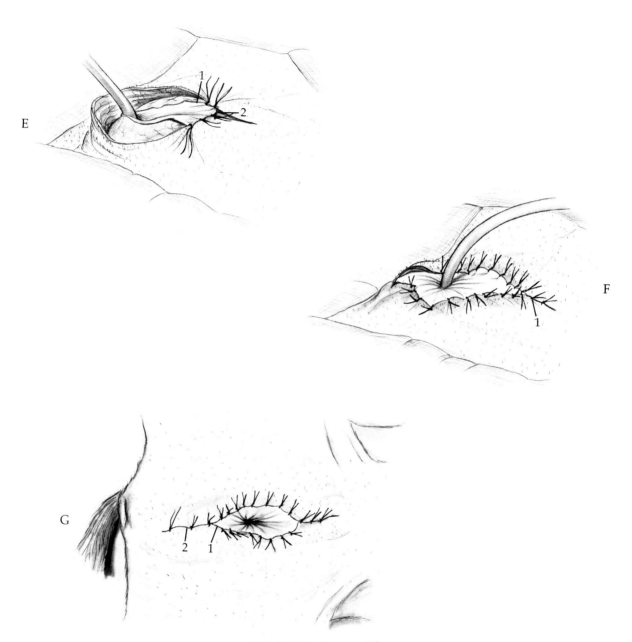

PLATE 58, cont'd

REFERENCES

Griener, T. P., and Greene, R. W.: Surgery of the urethra, J.A.A.H.A., p. 778, 1975.

Leighton, R. L.: Ablation of the penis and scrotum with a urethrostomy in the dog, J.A.A.H.A. **12**:661, 1976.

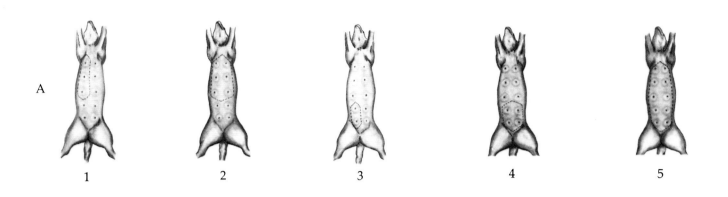

A

1   2   3   4   5

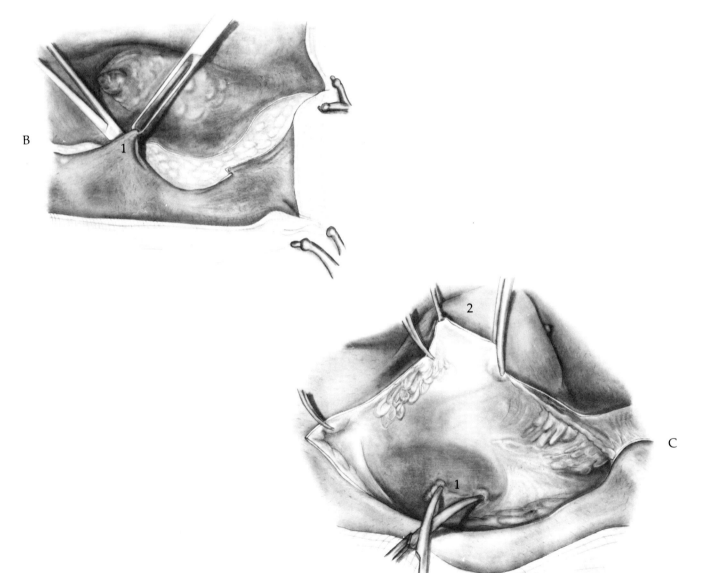

PLATE 59

Plate 60. Mastectomy

A The external inguinal ring *(1)* and the external pudendal vessels *(2)* are exposed by scissors dissection. The inguinal ring can be identified by palpating the femoral artery as it emerges from the body wall. The ring will be medial to this. Often the vaginal process may be palpated by inserting a finger beneath the gland and body wall. Care must be taken when exposing the vessels not to damage them.

B First the external pudendal artery is double ligated *(1)*, then the external pudendal vein *(2)*. The inguinal lymph node is located in the fatty tissue caudal to the ligated vessels *(3)*. If the vessels are ligated as they emerge from the ring and if the fatty and glandular tissue *(3)* is removed as a block, the external inguinal lymph node will be removed.

C The vessels are divided between the ligatures *(1)*. If a bilateral caudal mastectomy or a total mastectomy is to be performed, the incision, isolation, and ligation procedure is repeated on the opposite side. If a unilateral mastectomy is to be done, the medial incision is made after ligation of the vessels.

D Traction is placed on the mammary tissue in a cranial direction *(1)* and on the caudal skin flap in a posterior direction *(2)*. The glandular tissue is dissected free from the caudal skin flap, and bleeders are controlled by ligation. The procedure will undermine the caudal skin flap *(3)*. If only one side is to be removed, the glands are separated at the midline *(4)* prior to the dissection of the caudal aspect.

Once the caudal aspect of the gland is free, cranial traction is applied and the glands are separated from the body wall by scissors dissection. Bleeders from the skin and body wall are ligated. Large bleeders in the glandular tissue are clamped, but ligation of these is not necessary, since they will be controlled by cross clamping the gland.

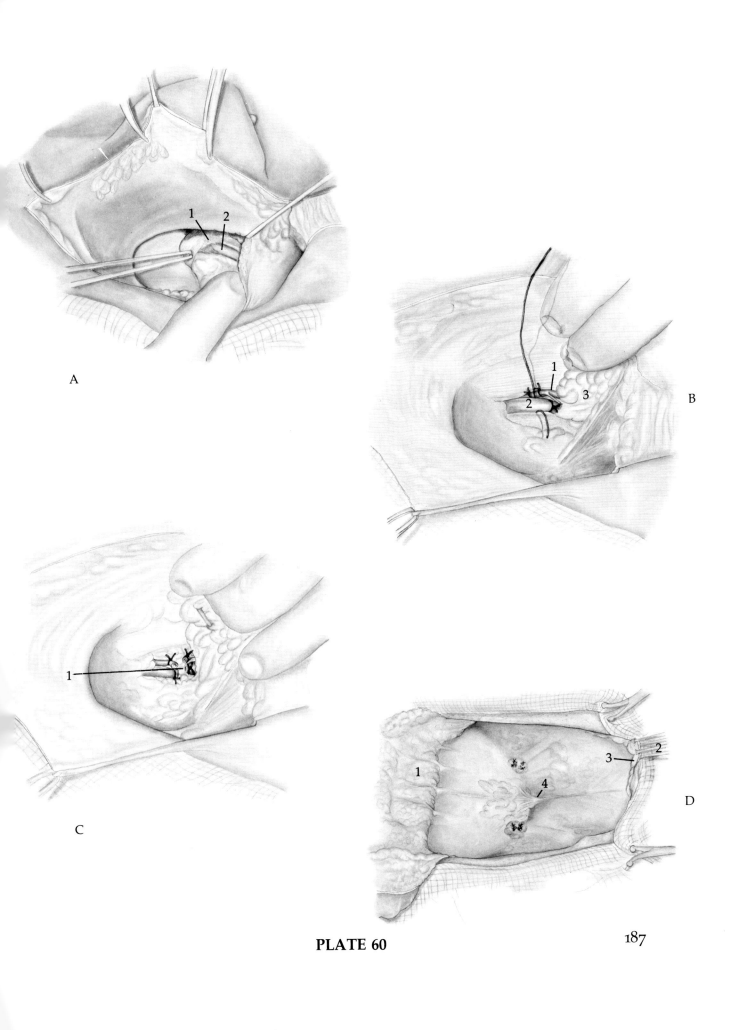

A

B

C

D

PLATE 60

Plate 61. Mastectomy

A The skin overlying the fourth and fifth glands just caudal to the third nipple is dissected free from the glandular tissue and undermined about 1 cm *(1)*. Two Carmalt forceps are placed across the glandular tissue. If only one side is to be removed, this side only is undermined and clamped. A simple continuous suture is started at the lateral aspect of the gland *(2)*. This is placed over a Carmalt forceps. One side is sutured, the Carmalt forceps is removed, and the suture is tightened *(4)*. The suture is continued over the Carmalt forceps *(3)* to the opposite side. Traction is applied to the beginning of the suture *(5)*.

B The second Carmalt forceps is removed, and the suture is tightened and tied *(1)*. Bleeding from the remaining glands has been controlled by this hemostatic suture. The suture pattern may be varied so that two sutures are used when bilateral removal is done. If one suture is utilized, it should be tightened at the midline. If one long suture is utilized and not tightened in the middle, the first side sutured may not pull tight enough to control bleeding. Note that the glandular suture line will retract behind the skin *(2)*. All bleeders remaining in the operative site are now ligated so that the field is dry before closure is begun. Cranial mastectomy is done in the same manner. The initial incisions are made as shown in Plate 59, *A* and *B*. The dissection is carried from cranial to caudal. During a cranial mastectomy, all bleeders are clamped and ligated as approached. Care should be taken to identify the perforating intercostal vessels and ligate these before cutting them. The remaining caudal glands are oversewn as described. If total mastectomy is performed, the dissection is continued from caudal to cranial. The perforating intercostal arteries should be identified and ligated before they are cut. These are visualized as the glands are reflected from the body wall. It should be remembered that the skin at the cranial aspect of the glands is not as mobile as the skin at the caudal aspect and that the initial incision should preserve as much skin as possible.

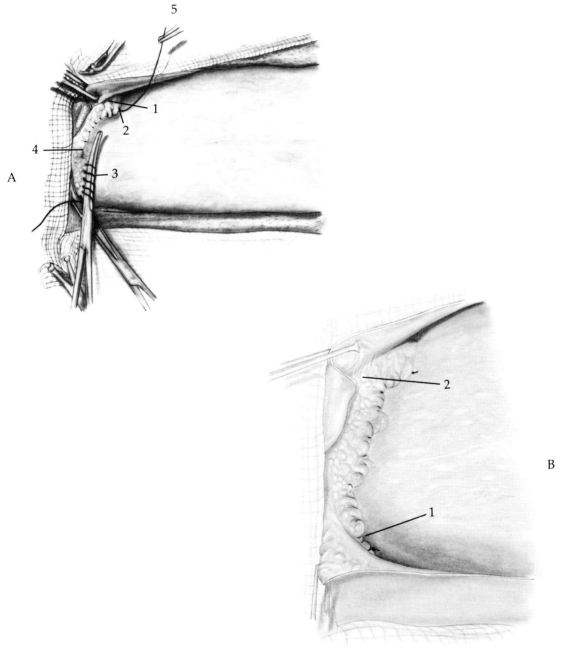

PLATE 61

Continued.

Plate 61. Mastectomy—cont'd

C Closure of the surgical site is accomplished with the same technique, whether the resection is total or partial. I prefer to use a Penrose drain, since this reduces the incidence of hematoma and seroma formation, especially with total mastectomy. However, some surgeons prefer not to drain. If tension on the skin suture line appears to be excessive, a stent pack may be used. This technique reduces the incidence of wound dehiscence and of suture pull out. The Penrose drains (1) are placed in the center of the incision. Two drains are used after a total mastectomy. One drain is placed from the cranial aspect of the incision to the level of the fourth mammary gland. The second is placed from the fourth mammary gland to the end of the incision. The drains should extend about 2 cm outside the skin. Holes may be placed in the drain but are not necessary. If the cranial glands are removed, only the cranial drain is placed. If the caudal glands are removed, only the caudal drain is placed. The subcutaneous tissue, if present, is closed with absorbable suture in a simple interrupted suture pattern (2). The area where the drains emerge is not tightly closed; this allows adequate drainage. Care is taken not to include the drains in the suture. It may be necessary to relax the tension on the hind legs to close the caudal aspect of the incision. Beginning at least 1.5 cm from the skin edge, tension sutures (3) for the stent pack are preplaced with a simple interrupted pattern of nonabsorbable suture. The sutures must not penetrate the subcutaneous tissue and must be left long enough to tie easily. The skin is closed with nonabsorbable sutures in a horizontal mattress (4) or simple interrupted suture pattern.

D The skin is completely closed except for the areas where the drains emerge. At these areas an opening of 1 to 1.5 cm is left, and a mattress suture loose enough to permit drainage and yet tight enough to hold the drains in position (1) is put in place. A roll of gauze is made from 3- by 3-inch sponges. This gauze roll (2) is placed on the incision site, and the tension sutures are tied over the roll and pulled tight enough to pucker the skin. The areas where the drains emerge are not tightly tied.

The stent pack is left in position for 5 days and then removed. The Penrose drains are left in position for 5 to 7 days or until they stop draining; during this time they should not be flushed. To remove the drains, simply cut the mattress sutures holding them and pull them out. The defects left by the drains are allowed to close by granulation.

To reduce the possibility of ascending infection, the patient should be kept off the cage floor by means of a rack. Appropriate antibiotics should be used. Appropriate methods of restraint should be used to prevent the patient's mutilating the wound.

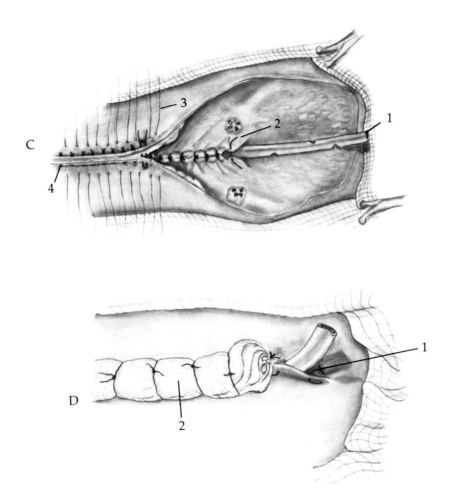

PLATE 61, cont'd

REFERENCES

Anderson, L. J., and Jarrett, W. F. H.: Mammary neoplasia in the dog and cat. II. Clinicopathological aspects of mammary tumor in the dog and cat, J. Small Anim. Pract. **7**:697, 1966.

Brodey, R. S., Fidler, I. J., and Howson, B. A.: The relationship of estrous irregularity, pseudopregnancy, and pregnancy to the development of canine mammary neoplasms, J. Am. Vet. Med. Assoc. **149**:1047, 1966.

Fidler, I. J., Abt, D. A., and Brodey, R. S.: The biological behavior of canine mammary neoplasms, J. Am. Vet. Med. Assoc. **151**:1311,1967.

Fidler, I. J., and Brodey, R. S.: Malignant mammary neoplasms, J. Am. Vet. Med. Assoc. **151**:710, 1967.

Owen, L. N.: Mammary neoplasia in the dog, J. Small Anim. Pract. **7**:703, 1966.

Schneider, R., Dorn, C. R., and Taylor, D. O. N.: Factors influencing canine mammary cancer and postsurgical survival, J. Natl. Cancer Inst. **43**:1249, 1969.

Silver, I. A.: Symposium on mammary neoplasia in the dog and cat. I. The anatomy of the mammary gland of the dog and cat, J. Small Anim. Pract. **7**:689, 1966.

25
Tracheal repair

Tracheal injury in the dog is usually the result of trauma. Since the damage generally occurs as the result of a dog fight, the repair has to be accomplished in a contaminated field.

The object of tracheal repair is to reestablish the continuity of the trachea without producing a stenosis. If any of the tracheal rings are fractured, they should be removed because they could cause a stenosis.

The cervical trachea is approached with a ventral midline cervical incision through the skin and subcutaneous tissue. The sternohyoid muscles are separated, exposing the trachea. If more exposure is necessary, the sternocephalic muscles may be separated at their attachment to the manubrium. Bleeders are controlled with ligatures of 3-0 chromic gut.

Plate 62.   Tracheal repair

A   The trachea has been exposed with a ventral midline incision. Care is taken to identify and preserve the recurrent laryngeal nerves if possible. If the area has been severely traumatized, these nerves are not easily visible. The right nerve runs on the right dorsolateral aspect of the trachea. The left nerve runs between the esophagus and trachea. Connective tissue has been dissected from the trachea and is being reflected medially and laterally *(1)*. This should be done carefully to preserve the recurrent laryngeal nerves. The tracheal lesion has been exposed. Note the connective tissue filling the tracheal lumen *(2)*.

B   The connective tissue has been removed from the tracheal defect, allowing the passage of a sterile endotracheal tube *(1)*. The tracheal muscle *(2)* may be seen. This is the only structure that is intact.

C   Simple interrupted sutures *(1)* of 3-0 chromic gut have been utilized to approximate a portion of the tracheal muscle.

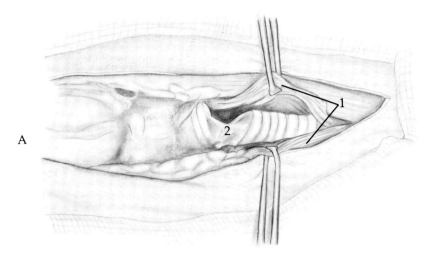

A

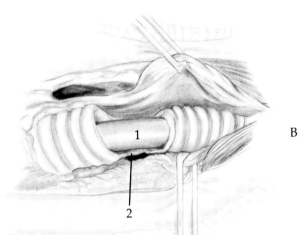

B

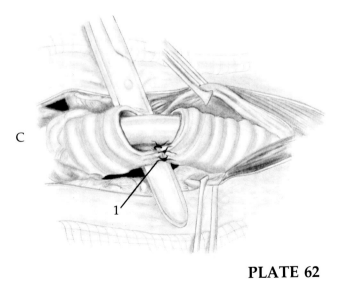

C

PLATE 62

Plate 63. Tracheal repair

A   Simple interrupted sutures *(1)* of nonabsorbable material have been placed through the cartilaginous rings. These are preplaced and then tied. Note that the tracheal rings are evenly approximated. If there is any overriding of the tracheal rings, a stenosis will result. The number of sutures used is determined by the diameter of the trachea. The tracheal rings should be brought into even apposition. Preplaced sutures *(2)* of 3-0 chromic gut have been placed around the tracheal sutures and into the reflected connective tissue *(3)*.

B   The preplaced sutures have been tied, drawing connective tissue over the tracheal defect. This connective tissue forms a seal over the tracheal repair and helps reduce air leakage from the repair. A Penrose drain *(1)* has been placed in the surgical site. This is necessary if the area is infected. The subcutaneous tissue *(2)* is closed with absorbable simple interrupted sutures, and the skin with nonabsorbable simple interrupted sutures.

The Penrose drain is removed when drainage from it stops. The animal is treated with antibiotics as determined by a culture taken at the time of surgery.

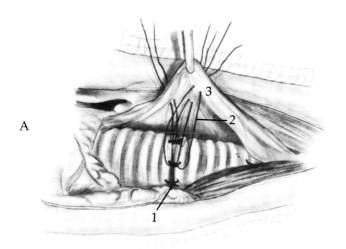

A

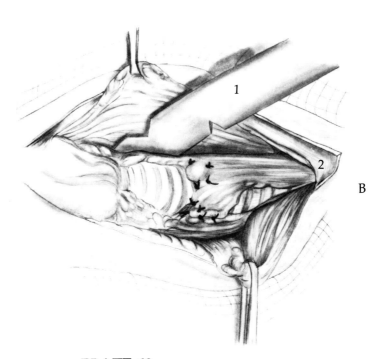

B

PLATE 63

26
Salivary mucocele and ranula

Cervical salivary mucoceles and ranulas are essentially the same type of lesion. They both result from the leakage of saliva through a defect in the mandibular or sublingual salivary systems. Saliva in the tissues produces a tissue reaction that results in the formation of a mucocele. In the case of a ranula, the mucocele is located ventral and lateral to the tongue and protrudes into the mouth on the involved side. When the mucocele is located ventrally, it is called a cervical salivary mucocele. Frequently a ranula and a mucocele may both be present; these may communicate.

The treatment of choice for salivary mucocele is to remove the involved mandibular and sublingual salivary glands and to drain the mucocele. The technique of marsupialization has been recommended for treatment of a ranula; however, most ranulas should be treated by salivary gland extirpation. Since it is often difficult to tell whether it is the mandibular or sublingual system that is involved and because the glands and ducts are in close anatomical proximity, both systems on the involved side are removed.

It should be emphasized that the surgical treatment of a salivary mucocele by extirpation of the salivary glands is less traumatic and simpler when it is done before any other form of therapy has been administered. The practice of draining and then injecting irritating agents into the mucocele generally does not eliminate the mucocele, but it does make the surgical treatment much more difficult.

A sialogram preoperatively *may* demonstrate which side is involved in the formation of a mucocele. However, if sialography is nondiagnostic, the side involved can usually be demonstrated at surgery.

The key aspects of the technique of salivary gland extirpation are a knowledge of the anatomy and a good control of hemorrhage to keep the surgical field clearly visible.

Plate 64. Salivary mucocele

A The dog is placed in the dorsal recumbent position, with a rolled up towel under its neck to maintain a horizontal position. An elliptical skin incision is made around the cervical mucocele, the size of the incision varying with the size of the mucocele; more skin will be removed with a larger incision. Only a minimal amount of skin should be removed with the cyst. It is better to remove excess skin when closing than to not have enough to close. The incision starts just cranial to the mucocele, encircles it, and continues distally over the jugular vein *(1)*.

B After the excess skin was removed, the mucocele was opened by a longitudinal incision, and its contents were evacuated. The cyst is now ready for examination. The trachea and larynx are located on the midline, and since the deepest portion of the cyst appears to be located on the right side of the trachea and larynx, the glands on the right side are the ones with the defect producing the mucocele. The same would be true for the left side. Many mucoceles will be multilocular, and it is necessary to open or palpate all pockets before determining on which side of the trachea most of the mucocele is located. Occasionally a small hole *(1)* may be visualized in the deepest aspect of the mucocele; this communicates with the involved glands or ducts. Note the mass of cystic tissue in the cranial portion of the cyst *(2)*. If the surgeon is not sure which side is involved, the cyst should be opened before the jugular is exposed. The incision to extirpate when only a ranula is present is begun at the external jugular vein just before it bifurcates, and it is carried cranially to the angle of the jaw, thereby exposing the salivary glands. Care is taken when incising over the external jugular vein not to inadvertently damage this structure. For good anatomical orientation it is important that the jugular vein be exposed in an area that is not involved either in the mucocele or in any inflammatory response associated with the mucocele. All bleeding should be controlled before proceeding.

C The external jugular vein *(1)* has been exposed. The area between the bifurcation of the lingual-facial *(2)* and maxillary *(3)* veins is exposed, and the mandibular and monostomatic sublingual glands *(4)* are palpated. These are generally deep at the lateral aspect of the mucocele. An occasional mucocele will lie deep in relationship to the glands, in which case the glands will be on the lateral aspect of the mucocele. The glands are located within a connective tissue capsule and are not easily visualized. In this illustration the mucocele *(5)* has not been incised in order to show anatomical relationships. The salivary glands are always deep to the jugular bifurcation. Occasionally, a cervical lymph node will be as large as the salivary glands; however, these nodes are usually superficial to the veins.

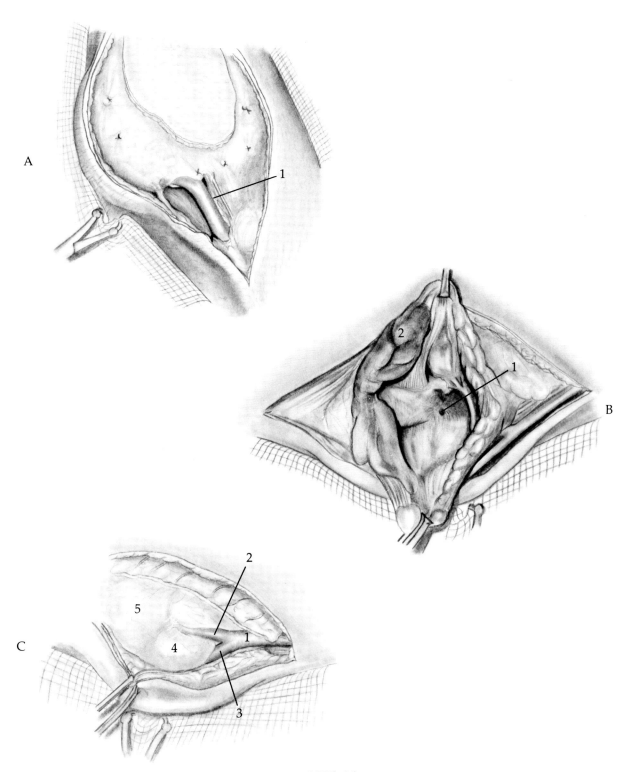

PLATE 64

Plate 65. Salivary mucocele

A A smaller mucocele *(1)* has been incised, and the mandibular and monostomatic portions of the sublingual salivary glands *(2)* are being dissected free from the capsule with gentle traction. As these glands are dissected, portions of the sublingual glands will be visualized along the duct.

B The mandibular and sublingual ducts *(1)* are dissected to the digastricus muscle *(2)*. This dissection requires cutting through the deeper portion of the mucocele *(3)*. If a mucocele has been previously manipulated, this portion of the procedure will be difficult, and profuse hemorrhage will be encountered. Care is taken not to remove excess tissue in this area, since this could result in damage to the ventral buccal nerve, producing a slight neurological deficit at the commissure of the mouth. This deficit is generally not noticeable except on close examination. The area *(4)* where the ducts pass under the digastricus muscle is digitally dissected so that the ducts are free for manipulation. The mandibular and sublingual ducts may be severed at this point by applying traction, working the ducts out from under the digastricus muscle, and ligating them. However, this will generally leave some sublingual tissue. If the location of the defect producing the mucocele has been positively identified, and if the mucocele is located lateral to the digastricus muscle, the aforementioned procedure would be sufficient. However, the location of most salivary mucoceles cannot be positively determined, and it could therefore involve the cranial portions of the sublingual glands. If a ranula is present, it is necessary to remove the cranial portions of the sublingual glands.

C A large salivary mucocele has been incised. The mandibular and sublingual glands *(1)* are dissected from their capsule. Note the deep portion of this mucocele *(2)*.

D The index finger *(1)* is carefully passed alongside the salivary ducts and under the digastric muscle *(2)* while maintaining traction of the salivary glands with an Allis tissue forceps *(3)*. The index finger *(1)* is passed through the floor of the cyst *(4)* medial to the digastric muscle. A closed Allis tissue forceps *(5)* is placed on the index finger.

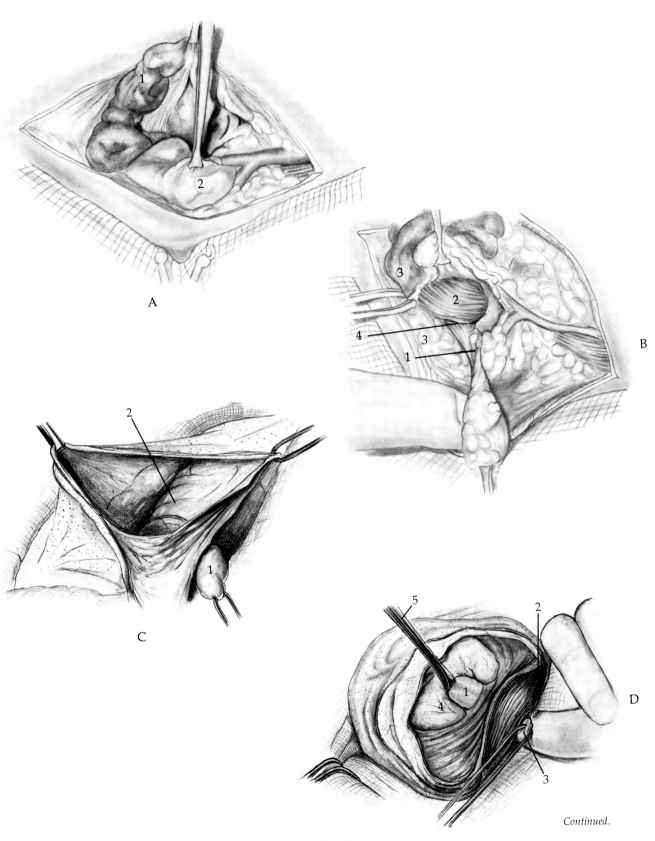

A

B

C

D

Continued.

PLATE 65

Plate 65. Salivary mucocele—cont'd

E   The Allis tissue forceps *(1)* is passed from medial to lateral under the digastricus muscle *(2)*. The salivary glands *(3)* are grasped by the forceps.

F   The salivary glands *(1)* are drawn by the Allis forceps from lateral to medial and emerge through the floor of the mucocele *(2)*.

G   The digastricus *(1)* and mylohyoid *(2)* muscles, with the floor of the cyst, are being reflected. The glands *(3)* and ducts *(4)* have been passed medially under the digastricus muscle. The external carotid *(5)* may be seen under the digastricus muscle, and care is taken when dissecting under the digastricus muscle not to damage this vessel. The lingual nerve *(6)* may be seen crossing the ducts.

H   The mylohyoid muscle and cyst floor *(1)* have been incised and are being reflected. Traction is being applied to the ducts *(2)*. The lingual nerve *(3)* has been gently dissected free from the ducts and reflected forward. A ligature *(4)* has been tied around the duct cranial to the sublingual glandular tissue *(5)*. The ducts are severed just caudal to the ligature. Note the hypoglossal nerve *(6)*, which is accompanied by the lingual vessels.

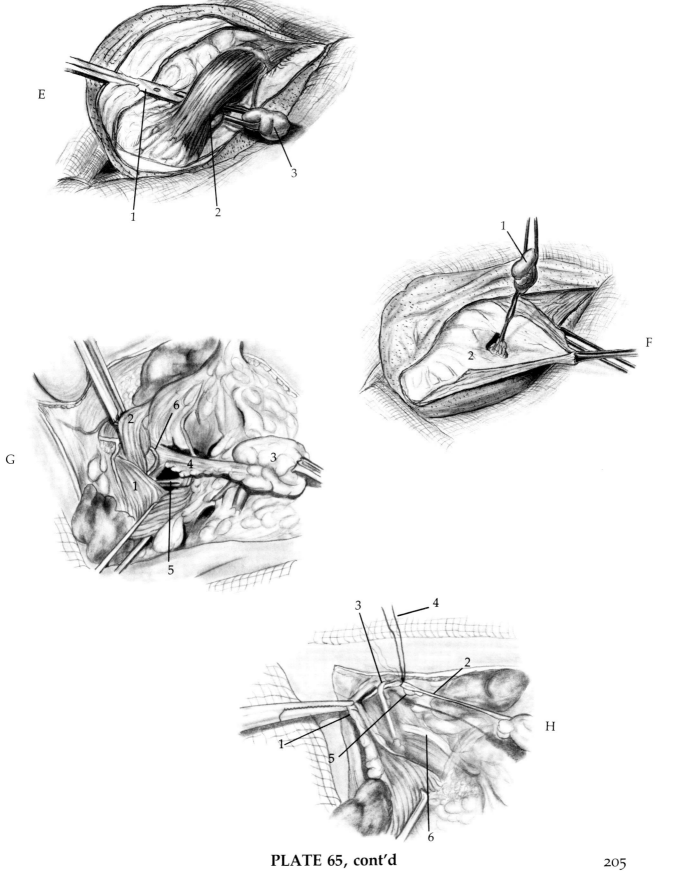

PLATE 65, cont'd

Plate 66.   Salivary mucocele

A   The ducts have been severed and the glands removed. The digastricus muscle *(1)* is being retracted laterally to demonstrate the lingual artery *(2)*, external carotid artery *(3)*, and facial artery *(4)*. The maxillary vein *(5)* is being retracted. The hypoglossal nerve is located next to the lingual artery but is not visible. Extreme care is taken when dissecting in this area because of the ease with which the vessels and nerves can be damaged. It must be emphasized that clear visibility must be maintained by controlling bleeding so that the surgeon has a dry clean field in which to work.

B   Two Penrose drains are used in the closure. The first drain *(1)* is placed in the area where the duct was ligated and divided and goes under the digastric muscle *(2)*. The second drain *(3)* is placed in the remaining mucocele. Both drains emerge in the portion of the wound that is most pendent when the dog is in a normal position. In a large dog the deep drain emerges in the middle of the wound, whereas in a smaller dog both drains may be brought out of the bottom of the wound.

C   The subcutaneous tissue is closed with simple interrupted sutures of 0 chromic gut, and a small opening is left for the drains *(1)*. The skin is closed in a simple interrupted or mattress suture pattern with nonabsorbable suture material. The area where the drains emerge from the skin is not closed, and the drains are fixed to the skin with a simple interrupted suture or mattress suture pattern that penetrates the drains.

The drains are left in position for 5 to 7 days or until drainage stops. The sutures are removed 7 to 10 days postoperatively. The mucocele may be cultured and appropriate antibiotics given.

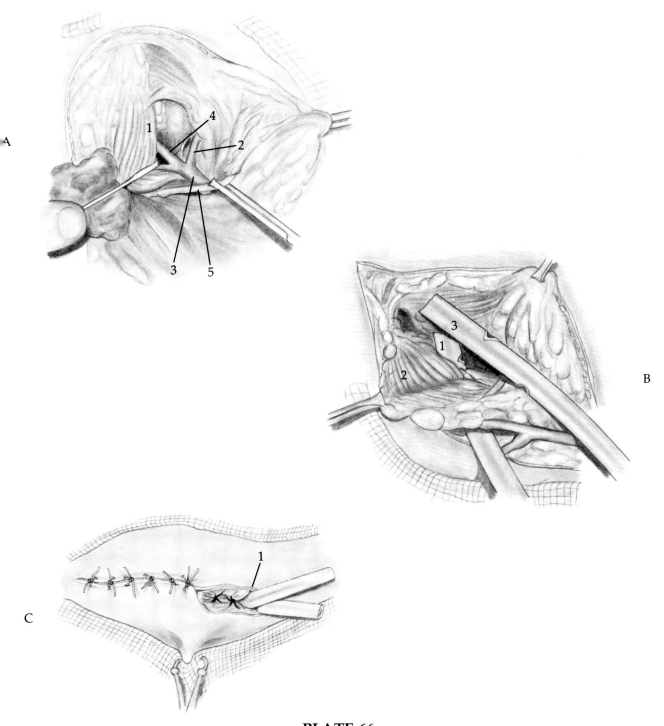

A

B

C

PLATE 66

REFERENCES

Glen, J. B.: Salivary cyst in the dog: identification of sublingual duct defects by sialography, Vet. Rec. **78**:488, 1966.

Hoffer, R. E.: Surgical treatment of salivary mucoceles, Vet. Clin. North Am. **5**:333, 1975.

Karbe, E., and Nielsen, S. W.: Canine ranulas, salivary mucoceles, and branchial cysts, J. Small Anim. Pract. **7**:625, 1966.

Spreull, J. S. A., and Head, K. W.: Cervical salivary cyst in the dog, J. Small Anim. Pract. **8**:17, 1967.

27
Resection of an elongated soft palate

Elongation of the soft palate is most commonly seen in brachiocephalic breeds. In these animals the condition is generally diagnosed when they are young. However, this condition can also be seen in older dogs that are not brachiocephalic in conformation.

Elongation of the soft palate interferes with respiration, since the palate blocks the larynx when the animal inspires, producing dyspnea. This is especially apparent following exercise, since it is not unusual for animals with an elongated soft palate to faint after exercising. Often in the brachiocephalic breed elongation of the soft palate will be associated with stenotic nares.

Surgical removal of the extra portion of the soft palate produces relief of these symptoms and generally improves the dog's exercise tolerance.

Plate 67. Soft palate resection

A The dog is placed in the sternal recumbent position with the head elevated. An endotracheal tube *(1)* is passed and fixed to the mandible. A mouth speculum *(2)* is inserted, and the mouth opened to its maximum extent. The larynx is examined by pulling the tongue forward. The soft palate *(3)* extends into the larynx, interfering with the closing of the epiglottis *(4)* with respiration.

B The excess soft palate should be removed so that when the larynx is in *normal* position the tip of the epiglottis just touches the remaining soft palate. If too much palate is removed, the dog will regurgitate nasally when eating or drinking. To determine the amount of palate to be removed, the tongue *(1)* is relaxed, placing the larynx in normal position. The tip *(2)* of the soft palate is grasped with an Allis tissue forceps and pulled forward. Two hemostats *(3)* are placed across the soft palate posterior to the Allis forceps at a level where the tip of the epiglottis just touches the forceps. These hemostats are not closed tightly until they are in exact position. The palate may be elevated to determine the exact position of the epiglottis. It may be necessary to remove the endotracheal tube to exactly position the hemostats. The tube should be reinserted before the soft palate is incised.

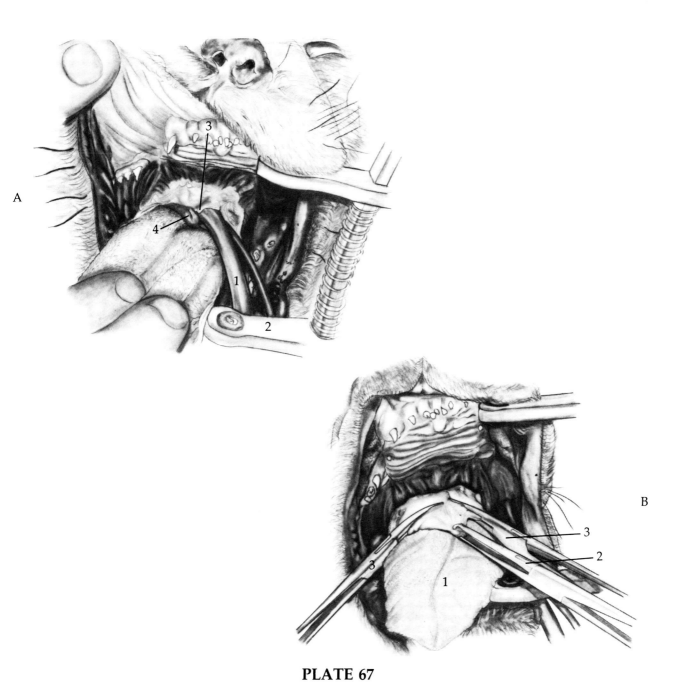

PLATE 67

A

B

211

Plate 68.   Soft palate resection

A   It should be remembered that approximately 1 mm of devitalized tissue will eventually be reabsorbed after resection because of the effects of the cautery and crushing by the hemostats. The excess soft palate is cut in front of the forceps *(1)* with electrocautery *(2)*. The hemostats are left in position a total of 7 minutes to allow clotting.

B   The cauterized tissue can be seen *(1)*. The tongue has been pulled forward, advancing the larynx. Note that in this position the epiglottis extends past the remaining soft palate *(2)*. If in doubt, the surgeon should remove less soft palate than he deems necessary. If, when the forceps are removed, too much soft palate remains, the forceps may be reapplied and the excess removed. An evaluation of the remaining soft palate is not made until traction on the tongue has been released and the larynx has been returned to a normal position. Moreover, the endotracheal tube should have been removed so that all the structures are in normal position before a decision is made as to whether sufficient soft palate has been removed.

C   The endotracheal tube has been removed, and traction on the tongue released. The tip of the epiglottis *(1)* extends slightly in front of the remaining soft palate *(2)*. Note that the laryngeal orifice, which was filled with tissue before surgery, is now open *(3)*. Since at least 1 mm of tissue will be reabsorbed from the soft palate, the tip of the epiglottis will just touch the remaining edge of the soft palate.

There is no bleeding from the cut edge of the palate. If excessive bleeding should occur, a simple continuous suture of 4-0 absorbable suture may be placed along the cut edge to control it.

The dog should receive corticosteroids, a diuretic, and antibiotics immediately after surgery. (Antibiotics should have been administered preoperatively as well.) This tends to reduce the inflammation and edema at the surgical site. The dog should be observed closely during the immediate postoperative period for evidence of swelling with respiratory distress or hemorrhage. If respiratory distress develops, a tracheotomy tube may be inserted. In older dogs tracheotomy may be done preoperatively to avoid postoperative upper respiratory obstruction problems. The dog should be kept on a soft diet for the first postoperative week.

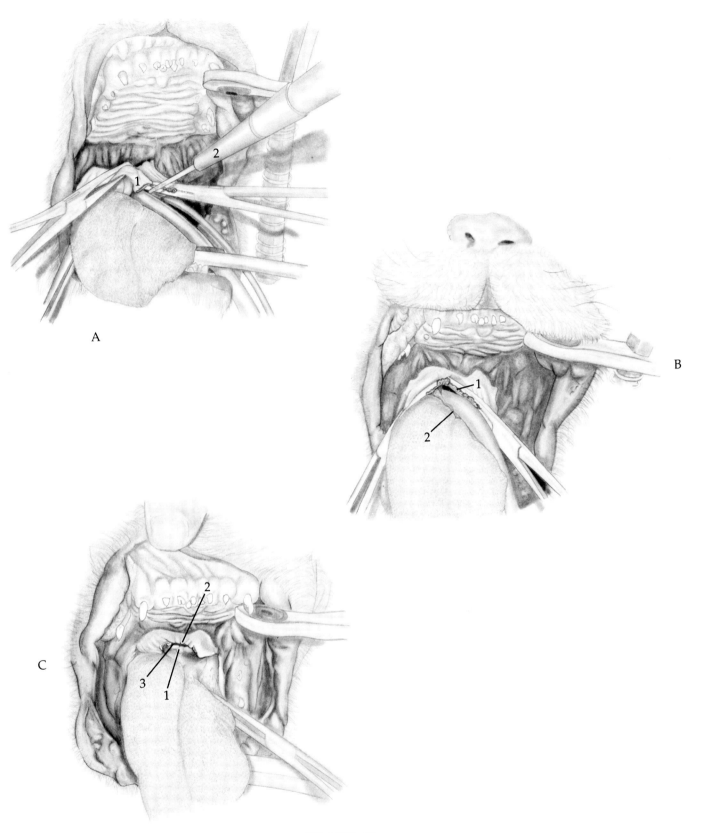

A

B

C

PLATE 68

28
Repair of inguinal hernia

Inguinal hernias occur most commonly in the older bitch but are occasionally seen in pups, both male and female. The technique described in this chapter applies to the repair of any inguinal hernia. In the male the closure of the caudal portion of the ring should be done carefully to prevent occlusion of the spermatic cord as it passes through the inguinal canal.

Plate 69. Inguinal hernia

    A   The appearance of an inguinal hernia in a bitch is shown.

    B   An incision is made through the skin and subcutaneous tissue just lateral to the mammary glands *(1)*. This incision should expose the hernial sac *(2)* but not enter it. Bleeders are controlled by ligation so that the operative field is dry.

    C   The hernial sac is entered by careful incision and completely opened *(1)*. The sac will generally contain fatty omental tissue *(2)*. Often in the older bitch it will contain the uterus. When opening the sac in the male, care must be taken not to damage the spermatic cord unless castration is anticipated.

    D   The hernial sac is dissected free from its attachment to the abdominal inguinal ring. Care is taken not to damage the pudendoepigastric trunk or the external pudendal vessels. The medial aspect of the sac has been dissected free, exposing the lateral border of the rectus abdominus muscle *(1)* and the fascia of the external abdominal oblique muscle *(2)*. A slit in the fascia of the external abdominal oblique forms the external inguinal ring (also called the subcutaneous ring). At this point, control of hemorrhage is important so that the various structures may be visualized. Traction is placed on the subcutaneous tissue to obtain better exposure of the area *(3)*. Note also that the skin and subcutaneous incision extends beyond the inguinal defect.

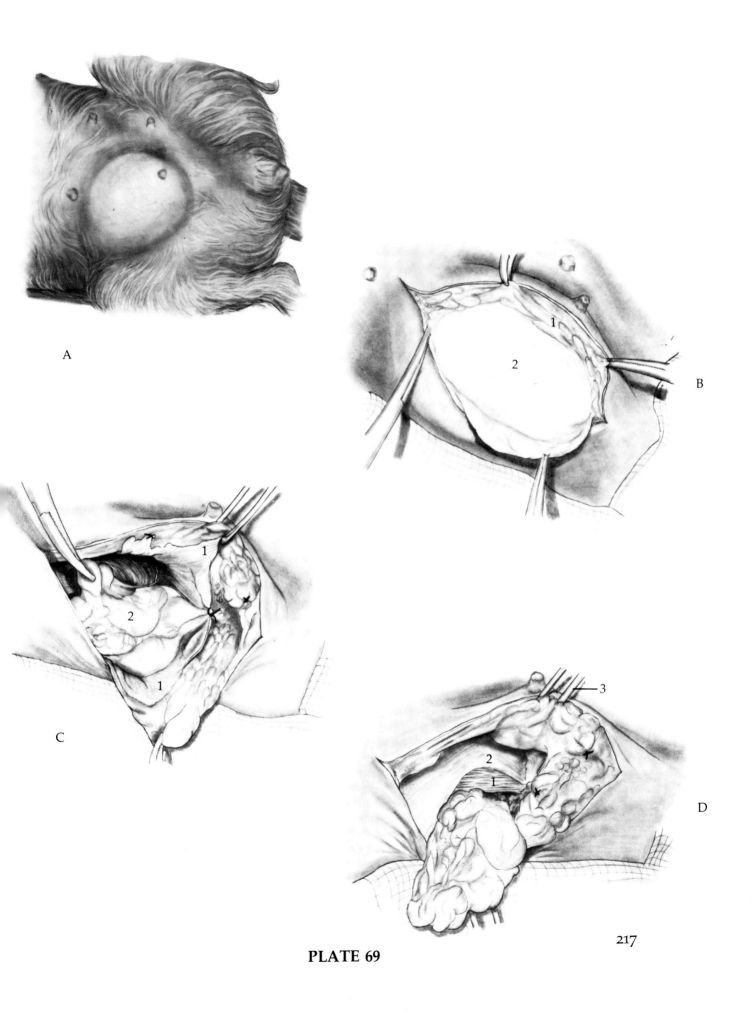

A

B

C

D

217

PLATE 69

Plate 70. Inguinal hernia

A   The fatty tissue in the sac has been retracted medially *(1)* to expose the cranial lateral aspect of the inguinal canal. The lateral aspect of the inguinal canal is formed by the pelvic tendon *(2)*, a fascial division of the aponeurosis of the external abdominal oblique. Lateral traction on the fascia of the external abdominal oblique *(3)* will demonstrate a tough fibrous band of tissue *(4)*, which can be seen and palpated deep in the lateral aspect of the canal.

B   The fatty tissue is being replaced into the abdomen *(1)*. The lateral border of the rectus abdominus muscle is elevated *(2)*. The cranial aspect of the inguinal canal has been incised 1.5 cm to give better exposure, thus exposing the fibers of the internal abdominal oblique *(3)*. Lateral traction on the pelvic tendon *(4)* demonstrates the firm fibrous band at the level of the internal ring *(5)*. Note the close proximity of this fibrous band of tissue to the deep femoral vessels *(6)*. The pudendoepigastric trunk *(7)* and the external pudendal vessels are also visualized *(8)*. These are generally covered by a fatty connective tissue and are not easily seen. The deep femoral artery arises from the external iliac artery, which, although not seen, is located slightly cranial to the fatty tissue *(1)*. These vessels must be palpated and identified before the hernia is closed. Enlarging the inguinal canal permits an ovariohysterectomy to be performed through the inguinal area. Some surgeons feel that an ovariohysterectomy should be performed to prevent recurrence of inguinal hernias in the bitch. In some cases the uterus may be trapped in the hernia, resulting in devitalization. If this occurs, ovariohysterectomy is necessary. In the male the spermatic cord will emerge from the caudal aspect of the ring. This should be carefully handled and protected.

C   The inguinal canal will be repaired with a two-layer technique. Care must be taken not to occlude the external pudendal vessels *(1)* or the spermatic cord. Either absorbable or nonabsorbable suture material may be used for the closure. A preplaced simple interrupted suture pattern is used for the first layer. The deep femoral and external iliac vessels are best protected by the surgeon's placing the index finger over them while placing the sutures. The first suture is passed through the lateral aspect of the rectus abdominus muscle *(2)*. The external oblique fascia *(3)* is not included. The suture should include the transversalis fascia *(4)*. Medial traction is applied to the subcutaneous tissue *(5)* and lateral traction to the pelvic tendon *(6)*.

D   Traction is applied to the pelvic tendon *(1)*, and the needle is carefully inserted through the fibrous band at the deep portion of the canal *(2)*. Placement of the needle should be extremely exact at this point in the suture pattern. The deep femoral vessels and external iliac vessels are protected with the surgeon's finger. The needle is placed in close proximity to the deep femoral vessels at this point.

218

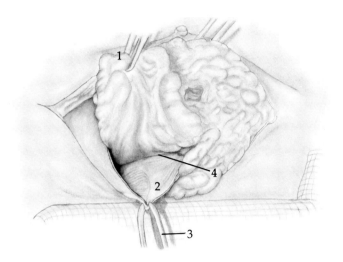

A

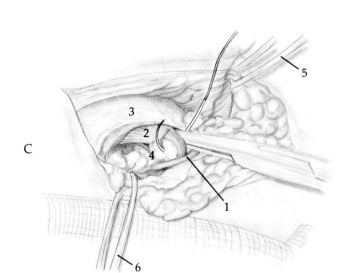

C

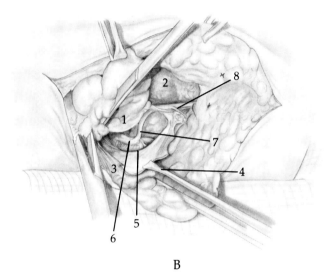

B

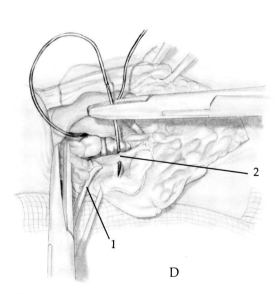

D

PLATE 70

Plate 71. Inguinal hernia

A All the sutures necessary to properly close the ring are placed before any are tied. Note that the caudal portion of the ring is loosely closed to permit free passage of the external pudendal vessels or spermatic cord if present. Note also how the sutures pass through the base of the pelvic tendon *(1)*.

B The sutures have been tied, thus closing the abdominal ring. The lateral border of the rectus abdominus has been apposed to the deep portion of the pelvic tendon. The internal abdominal oblique muscle, which was severed to enlarge the canal, has been closed with a simple interrupted suture pattern.

C The subcutaneous or external ring is closed with simple interrupted sutures. The area of external abdominal oblique fascia that was previously incised to enlarge the ring should be closed. Note that the suture goes through the muscle fascia and pelvic tendon only.

D The external ring has been closed. Note that the caudal aspect of the ring has not been occluded.

The subcutaneous tissue is closed with absorbable simple interrupted sutures. All dead space is eliminated to prevent seroma formation. The skin is closed with a simple interrupted pattern of nonabsorbable suture. If the hernia is bilateral, the other side is repaired before the skin is closed. If excessive dead space is present, a Penrose drain may be used.

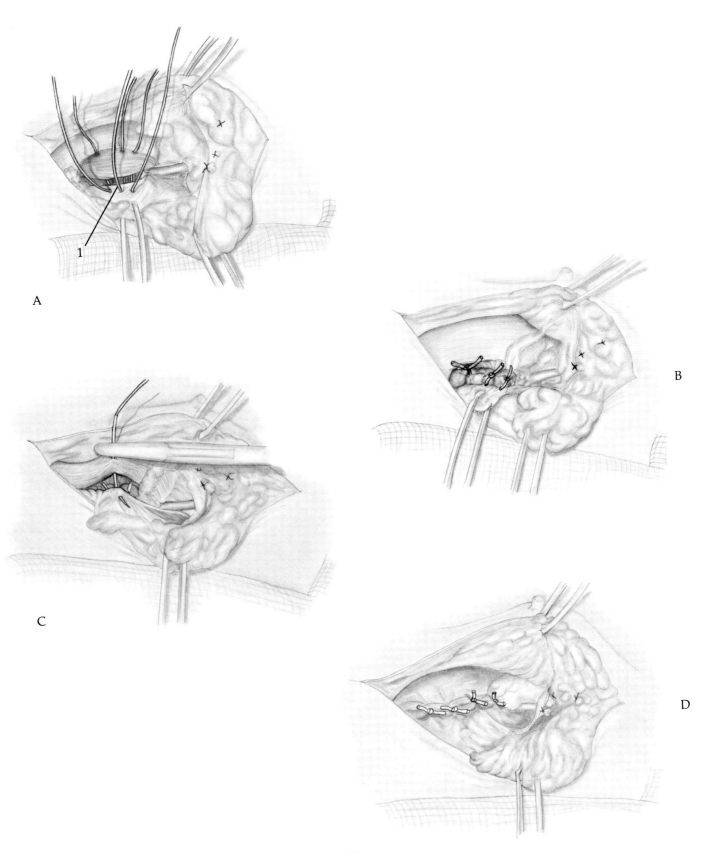

A

B

C

D

PLATE 71

29
Perineal hernia repair

Perineal hernias occur most commonly between the levator ani and the rectum and occasionally between the levator ani and coccygeus muscle. Generally these hernias contain a mass of fat, but they may also contain the urinary bladder and the prostate gland. Occasionally, if the the hernia has been present for a long period of time, the hernial sac may contain fluid and be mistaken on palpation for the bladder. On rectal palpation a pouching of the rectum into the hernial sac can be felt.

Perineal hernias may be bilateral or unilateral. Generally, if there is a unilateral hernia, careful palpation will reveal a weakness on the opposite side. In some cases, repair of the unilateral hernia with castration will prevent the development of the hernia on the weakened side. Bilateral hernias may also show a definite weakness ventrally, which makes their repair more difficult.

Bilateral hernias may be repaired simultaneously, depending on the condition of the patient and how the patient responds during the surgical procedure. It must be noted that bilateral hernial repair can result in fecal incontinence if bilateral damage occurs to the pudendal nerves or their branches. Knowledge of the anatomy and careful control of hemorrhage to maintain good visualization of the surgical site will enable the surgeon to identify and protect the triad of pudendal nerve, internal pudendal artery, and vein.

Many surgeons recommend that castration follow the repair of a perineal hernia to prevent recurrence. However, there has been one study that suggest that castration will not affect the recurrence of a perineal hernia.

The basic technique of repair is the reconstruction of the muscular diaphragm alongside the rectum. This is done by suturing the levator ani and coccygeus muscles to the internal obturator muscle and the external anal sphincter.

Plate 72. Perineal hernia

A A bilateral perineal hernia presents as a bilateral pouching on either side of the rectum. The bulge becomes more prominent with abdominal straining. If the hernial sac contains the bladder, the bladder is replaced into the abdomen by digital pressure after the operative site is clipped. In some cases it may be necessary to catheterize the bladder before it can be replaced. An enema may be administered 12 hours prior to surgery if the distal colon contains a large mass of feces. The anus is closed with a tight purse-string suture. If the fecal material is soft, two sutures should be used. The dog is placed with the hind legs over the elevated well-padded end of an operating table. The tail is elevated and fixed in this position. The incision *(1)* is begun 1 cm lateral to the tail head and 1 to 2 cm above it. The incision is curved laterally around the anus and then medially, staying about 1 cm from the midline. The incision should penetrate only the skin. Bleeders are controlled with ligatures of 3-0 chromic gut.

B The hernial sac is carefully opened by scissors dissection from the level of the caudal border of the superficial gluteal muscle to the level of the pubis. The hernial sac usually contains a mass of fat *(1)* that is adhering to connective tissue, thus obscuring the perineal muscles.

C The hernial sac may contain the urinary bladder *(1)*.

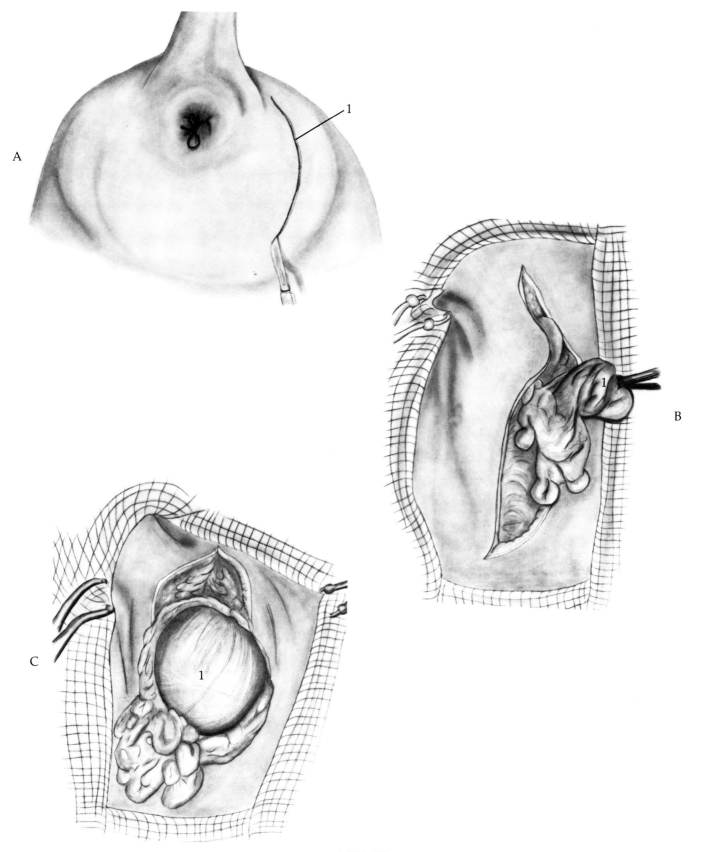

A

B

C

PLATE 72

Plate 73.   Perineal hernia

A   The hernial sac may contain an enlarged prostate gland *(1)*, in which case the bladder usually will be full. The urinary bladder is expressed, and the bladder and prostate gland are gently replaced into the abdominal cavity. The fatty adhesions are gently separated from their attachments by blunt dissection. Extreme care is taken during this procedure because the fat obscures the pudendal triad, and it is at this point that damage may occur. All bleeders should be ligated so that a dry, clear operative field is maintained.

B   This illustration demonstrates the normal anatomy of a dog. The colon *(1)*, external anal sphincter *(2)*, levator ani and coccygeus muscles *(3)*, internal obturator muscle *(4)*, and pudendal triad *(5)* are all visible. The coccygeal muscles in a dog with a perineal hernia are generally atrophied, and the division between the levator ani and coccygeus muscles is difficult to see. However, the hernia generally occurs between the colon and the levator ani muscle. Generally the coccygeal muscle mass is a combination of both. The pudendal triad is located on the internal obturator muscle. It emerges between the coccygeus muscle and the area *(6)* where the superficial gluteal muscle crosses the sacrotuberous ligament, which can be palpated. The nerve and vessels pass in a medial direction across the internal obturator muscle, where it gives off the caudal rectal nerves and vessels *(7)*. Often the fatty mass of the hernial sac will surround the triad. Careful dissection is necessary to preserve the pudendal triad, as well as the caudal rectal nerve and vessels.

C   The dissected fat may be removed or replaced into the abdominal cavity with an Allis tissue forceps *(1)* and sponge. The defect between the rectum and the coccygeal muscles should also be cleaned of this fat. After the fat is replaced (or removed), the structures to be sutured may be visualized. These are the levator ani and coccygeus muscles *(2)*, the external anal sphincter *(3)*, and the internal obturator muscle *(4)*. The pudendal triad *(5)* should be protected so that a suture is not inadvertently passed around or through it. Generally the levator ani muscle is not specifically seen, since this is often partially destroyed by the hernia.

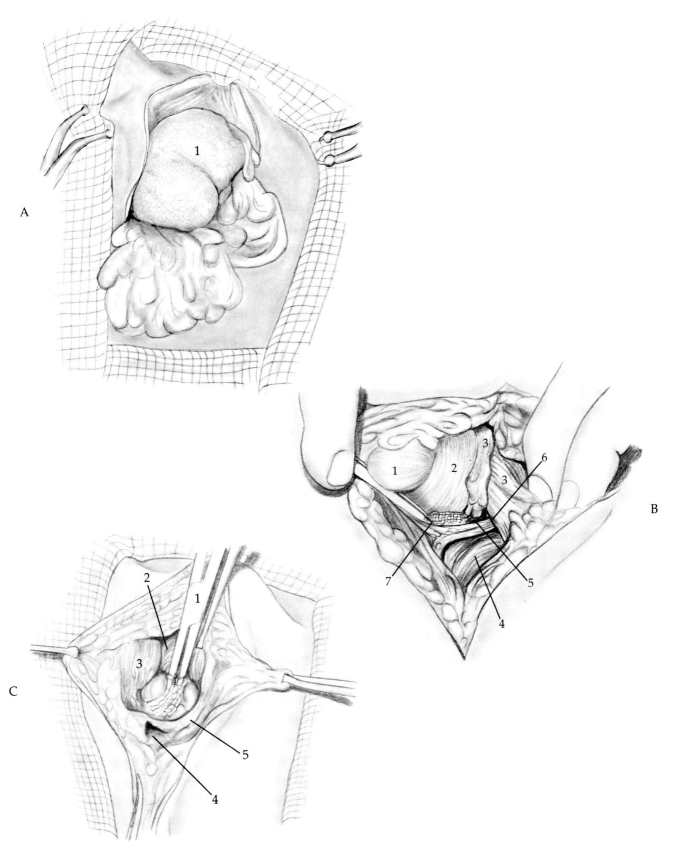

A

B

C

PLATE 73

227

Plate 74. Perineal hernia

A The pelvic diaphragm is reconstructed with a preplaced suture technique of 1 chromic gut. Stainless steel sutures may be used if the surgeon desires. If the defect is large, it is generally closed as a triangle. Care must be taken when suturing not to include the pudendal triad (1) in any of the sutures. The dorsal aspect of the defect is closed by placing sutures (2) through the external anal sphincter (3) and into the coccygeal muscles (4). If the coccygeus muscle is atrophied, the sutures may include some of the superficial gluteal muscles and sacrotuberous ligament for added strength. Care should be taken when suturing the sacrotuberous ligament because it is possible to damage the sciatic nerve, which is cranial to the ligament. The lateral aspect of the defect is closed by placing sutures (5) from the coccygeal muscles to the internal obturator muscle (6). The ventral aspect of the defect is closed by putting sutures (7) through the external anal sphincter (3) and the internal obturator muscle (6). Note that these sutures are placed caudal to the pudendal triad (1).

B If there is a ventral aspect to the defect, sutures (8) are placed medially to fix the ventral aspect of the external sphincter (3) to the internal obturator muscle (6), being careful to avoid the urethra. All the sutures are in place, and the final suture (9) is being placed from the coccygeal muscles (4) to the external anal sphincter (3). To summarize suture placement, sutures 2 and 9 attach the external anal sphincter to the coccygeal muscles, suture 5 attaches the coccygeal muscles to the internal obturator muscle, and sutures 7 and 8 attach the external anal sphincter to the internal obturator muscle. Tension is put on these sutures, and the repair palpated. If there is any defect in the closure, additional sutures are placed.

C The sutures are tied, completing the reconstruction of the pelvic diaphragm. The subcutaneous tissue is closed with simple interrupted sutures of 0 chromic gut. It may be necessary to use two subcutaneous layers in some dogs.

The skin is closed with nonabsorbable sutures in a simple interrupted or mattress suture pattern. If bilateral hernia repair is necessary, the opposite side is repaired before the skin is closed.

After the hernia is repaired, the dog is immediately castrated. The purse-string suture is then removed. The dog is kept on a soft diet for 7 postoperative days, and the sutures are removed in 10 days or when healing has occurred. Appropriate antibiotics may be used.

228

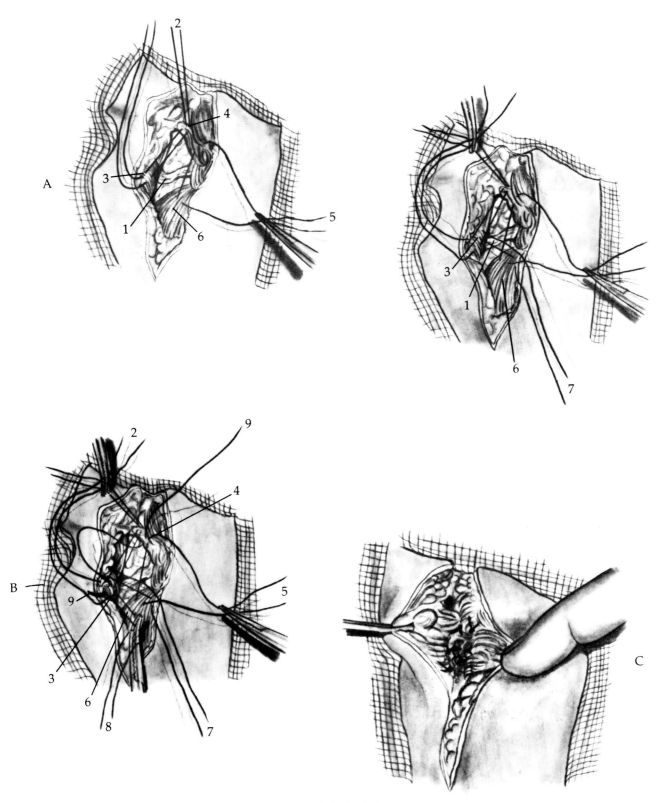

PLATE 74

REFERENCES

Burrows, C. F., and Harvey, C. E.: Perineal hernia
in the dog, J. Small Anim. Pract. **14**:315, 1973.
Pettit, G. D.: Perineal hernia in the dog, Cornell
Vet. **52**:261, 1962.

INSTRUMENTATION

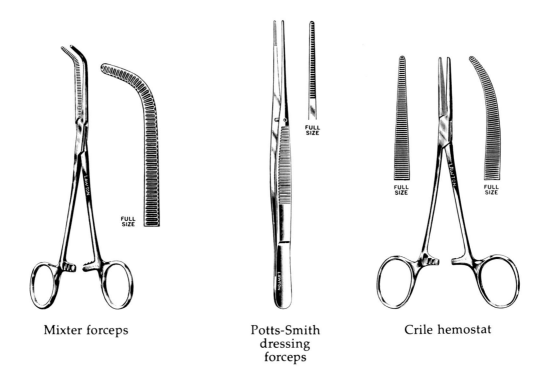

Mixter forceps

Potts-Smith
dressing
forceps

Crile hemostat

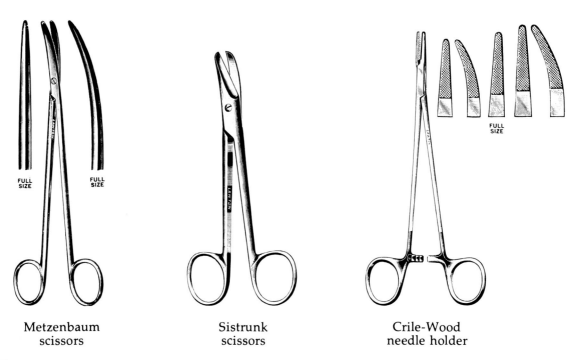

Metzenbaum
scissors

Sistrunk
scissors

Crile-Wood
needle holder

Illustrations courtesy the Lawton Co., Inc., Moonachie, N.J.; from Surgical instrument catalog, 1970.

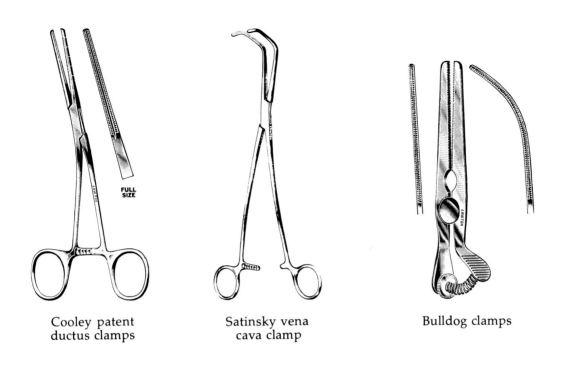

Cooley patent
ductus clamps

Satinsky vena
cava clamp

Bulldog clamps

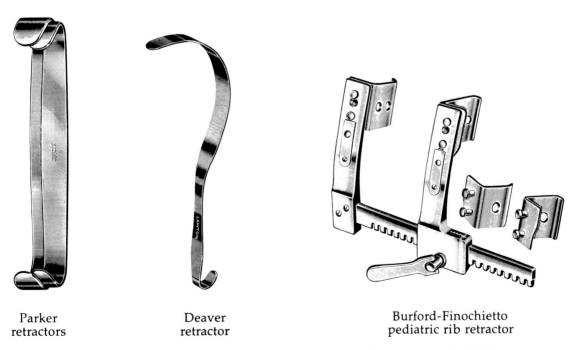

Parker
retractors

Deaver
retractor

Burford-Finochietto
pediatric rib retractor

Illustrations courtesy The Lawton Co., Inc., Moonachie, N.J.; from Surgical instrument catalog, 1970.

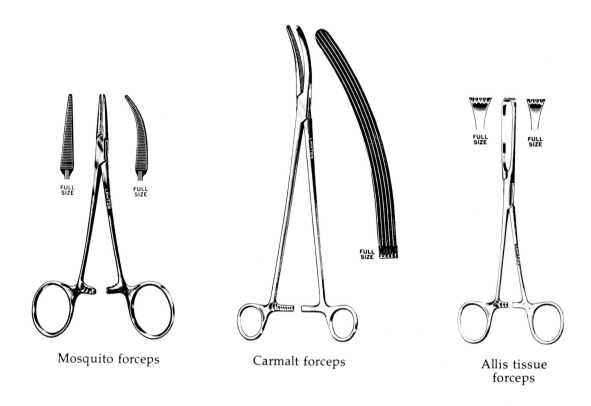

Mosquito forceps

Carmalt forceps

Allis tissue
forceps

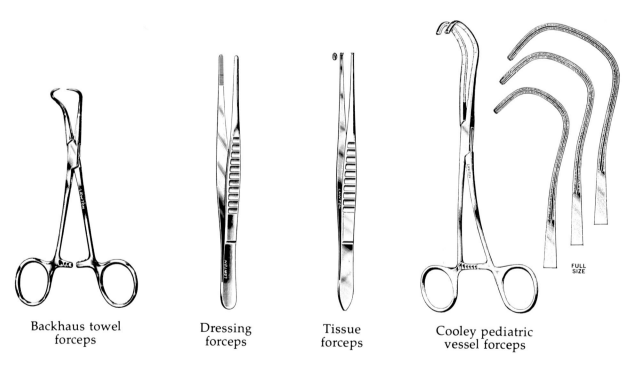

Backhaus towel
forceps

Dressing
forceps

Tissue
forceps

Cooley pediatric
vessel forceps

Illustrations courtesy the Lawton Co., Inc., Moonachie, N.J.; from Surgical instrument catalog, 1970.

234

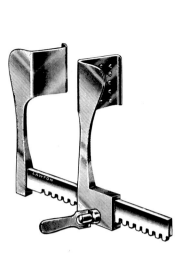

Reinhoff-Finochietto
rib spreader*

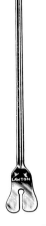

Grooved
director*

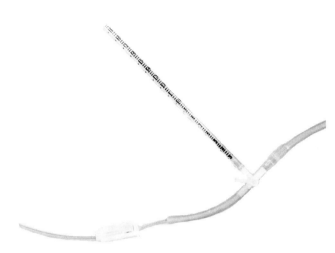

Central venous pressure
monitoring setup †

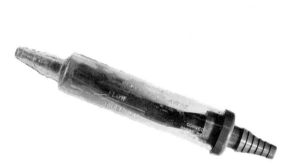

Heimlich valve ‡

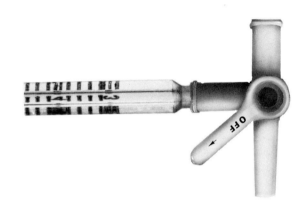

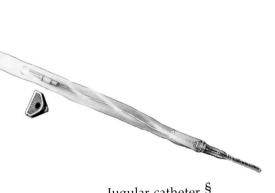

Jugular catheter §

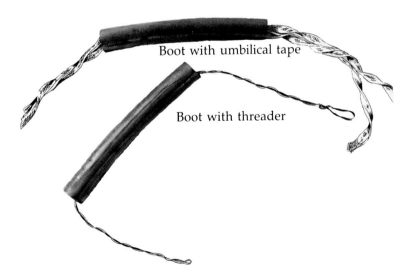

Boot with umbilical tape

Boot with threader

*Courtesy The Lawton Co., Inc., Moonachie, N.J.; from Surgical instrument catalog, 1970.
†Pharmaseal Laboratories, Glendale, Calif.
‡Bard-Parker Co., Division of Becton, Dickinson, Inc., Rutherford, N.J.
§Deseret Pharmaceutical Co., Sandy, Utah.

235

BIBLIOGRAPHY

Archibald, J., editor: Canine surgery, ed. 2, Santa Barbara, Calif., 1974, American Veterinary Publications, Inc.

Kirk, R. W., editor: Current veterinary therapy, small animal practice, Philadelphia, 1971, W. B. Saunders Co., vols. III, IV, and VI.

Leonard, E. P.: Fundamentals of small animal surgery, Philadelphia, 1968, W. B. Saunders Co.

Miller, M. E., Christensen, G. C., and Evans, H. E.: Anatomy of the dog, Philadelphia, 1964, W. B. Saunders Co.

Osborne, C. A., Low, D. G., and Finco, D. R.: Canine and feline urology, Philadelphia, 1972, W. B. Saunders Co.

Schwartz, S. I., editor: Principles of surgery, New York, 1969, McGraw-Hill Book Co.

INDEX